Trumpet of Clay

The Jerry Franks Story

Trumpet of Clay

The Jerry Franks Story

by Toni Morehead

Wesley Press
Indianapolis, Indiana

Published by Wesley Press
Indianapolis, Indiana 46250
Printed in the United States of America
ISBN 0-89827-051-0

Contents

Thank You

A special thank you to doctors, nurses, students, musicians and the friends and family of Jerry Franks for their contributions through written, phone, and personal interviews.

Toni Morehead

Foreword

Among the many talented and diverse individuals I have met in my over 30 years in public life, I'm hard pressed to name anyone who has been as personally inspirational to me as Indiana's own Jerry Franks. Jerry is certainly that special kind of human being that far too few of us have the opportunity to meet in a lifetime.

He has not only personally and professionally triumphed over severe adversities and physical hardships, he has emerged from each battle better and stronger of character than before. He has never lost his enthusiasm for life, his commitment to hard work nor his deep abiding faith in the Almighty.

Beyond this, perhaps his greatest legacy is the young men and women he has helped develop not only into fine musicians, but into exemplary citizens as well.

Despite all his obvious professional talents as one of the world's premier trumpet players, he has declined numerous opportunities for fame in favor of sharing his craft and zest for life with ambitious young musicians. It is certainly fair to say that each day Jerry Franks lives the credo, "Service above self."

It is an honor to call him my friend.

Otis R. Bowen, M.D.
Secretary of Health
and Human Services,
former governor of Indiana

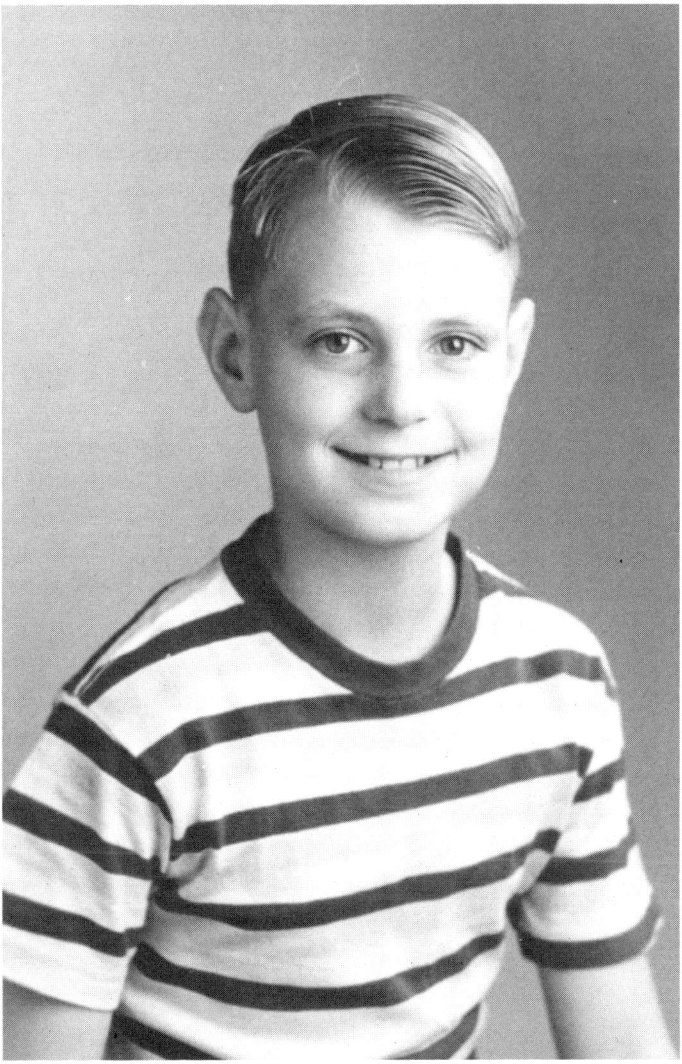

Jerry Franks: A healthy 13 year old (1951)

But they that wait upon the Lord shall renew their strength; they shall mount up with wings as eagles; they shall run and not be weary; and they shall walk, and not faint (Isa. 40:31). Jerry's "life verse" chosen when he was 12 years old.

Chapter 1

Blind!

Easter morning 1978. 7:00 a.m.

Jerry Franks came up from sleep slowly, trying to remember where he was. He heard the mumble of voices from somewhere in the house, but the female voice was not that of his wife, Dottie; the male voice did not belong to one of his sons. Coffee was brewing; they must be getting breakfast.

Oh, yes. Don and Donna Bechtel. He was at the Bechtel house. If he hadn't stayed up late talking to Don he might be able to think better.

But the talk had been good, catching up on what Don was doing since he'd graduated from Grace College and gone on to teaching. It was always satisfying to hear from former students, to know that he'd helped them become good musicians and teachers.

The clink of spoon against dish reminded Jerry that he had more to do than lie in bed in a half stupor; there was a busy day of concerts ahead. A morning service in the South Bend church, an afternoon concert in the Osceola church and lots of lively college kids to herd around in between. And good food! The church ladies always brought out their best, from the best cooks.

Jerry blinked slightly scratchy eyelids and looked up at the ceiling.

Why was it so dark? . . . Was it earlier than he thought? Why were Don and Donna up if it was so dark? . . . Perhaps his eyes were not accustomed to the light, or they were blurred with sleep.

He blinked several times more, trying to clear his vision, but all he could see was a gray haze. He could not see the ceiling! Lazy relaxation disappeared. Sickness! His stomach was a knotted illness, as realization washed over him. He was not going to see the ceiling. He was blind! But the doctor had said he wouldn't go blind.

He'd had trouble with his vision the previous December as he was returning from an appearance in Kansas, and on a Christmas trip back to Pennsylvania. Each time his sight had returned and the doctor had said he wouldn't go blind. The doctor was wrong!

But maybe he'd known even then that the doctor could be wrong. Why else had he memorized 55 method books – "just in case"? What else could he have done? He had to teach 90 students and direct the Dimensions in Brass, and he had to have a way to continue making a living.

Whoa! he said to himself. Let's think positive. If your sight came back before, maybe it will this time too.

He didn't believe that. The other times his vision had been hazy or shortened. This time he could tell if his eyes were directed on something bright or dark, nothing more. The knotted illness was back in his stomach. Help, Lord!

There was so much to do. He and the Grace College Dimensions in Brass had just begun a spring tour, two weeks of concerts in three states. He had 25 concerts to conduct, solos to play. If he couldn't continue, the tour would have to be canceled.

He'd been told what diabetes might do to eyes and circulation. Hemorrhage in the eyes – that was what caused blindness. Blindness! No, please, Lord. Help me!

Jerry lay still, remembering some of the scriptures he'd known since childhood. God promised to be a refuge and strength, a help in time of trouble. Yes. God was unchanging, loving. Unchanging in His loving, He would help. God help me!

Suddenly it was there. How could he ever describe it? Not lightning from heaven or messages on the mirror, just peace. Floating on calm waters. A feeling that everything would be all right.

Peace. God promised peace. Now Jerry knew the word. Like a baby learning about the textures around him, Jerry felt, tested, *savored* God's peace. It was now part of him, to summon up when he needed the knowledge.

"Be all right" was the promise. Not sight, not the name of a doctor or a procedure, but an assurance that freed his mind to think about immediate problems: how was he going to manage the concert at 9:30?

Well, one thing was sure, he would need the help of Don and Donna. And since they could see, whether he could or not, it might be good to get dressed. He smiled to himself. He didn't want to shock them with two startling revelations at once!

Groping in a circle from the bed, he found the suitcase he'd placed on the floor the night before.

Probably mess up the whole thing, he thought, undo all Dottie's neat packing trying to find a shirt. Dottie. How would his blindness affect her? She'd been his girl since they were children, and then a caring wife who supported his belief in God's plan for their lives.

Just then his groping fingers touched the stiff edges of an envelope. He extracted it from beneath some shirts and held it a moment as a new realization of blindness washed over him. Dottie had put in an Easter card to surprise him and he wouldn't be able to read it.

He ran his fingers over the surface of the envelope and swallowed hard, trying to dispel the tightness in his throat. Blindness meant he would never again read her words of affection.

After pulling on a pair of pants, Jerry stood where he was and called to Donna. He couldn't remember much of the room, so he thought it best to stay put.

"Jerry?" Donna's questioning voice came through the door.

"C'mon in, Donna."

Jerry heard the movement of the latch and the scuff of her slippers on the floor. Then the footsteps stopped. She did not speak.

"I can't see, Donna. I'm going to need help."

There was only a tick of time until she spoke. "What can I do?"

Donna, who had roomed with Dottie and Jerry when she was a student at Grace, helped him orient himself to room and bathroom, laid towel, soap and washcloth across the lavatory and directed his hand to them. Then she left, closing the door quietly behind her.

With each everyday action, Jerry found a new realization to ponder. Blindness meant struggling to find the front and back and up and down of things, and still finishing with shirts and coats buttoned crooked. Blindness meant wasted moments while he groped for slippery soap and struggled with globs of toothpaste that found their way to everything but the toothbrush. And his electric razor, which had been such a friend in a busy schedule, became a buzzing gremlin that gobbled up sideburns before he knew it. One thing he knew for sure, blindness would be a challenge.

When Jerry entered the kitchen he took with him the quip-cracking, impish sense of humor that had always made people groan and then smile in spite of themselves.

"Boy, Donna," he said, "you must have cooked something bad for supper last evening, 'cause I went blind last night!"

Haltingly, feeling with his toe, his arms extended, he shuffled through the doorway. Then he stopped, too unsure to continue.

The people around the table were stunned. Fred Bechtel, Don's brother, was a member of the Dimensions in Brass and had stayed overnight too. Don and Donna, though they knew of the blindness, did not know its severity or the care and concentration with which Jerry reached for each step and guidepost. Blind overnight. How could it happen to Jerry? And how could he take it so calmly?

"Hey, do I get some breakfast, you guys?"

The Bechtels relaxed. Jerry was the same old Jerry. It would be easier if they could make jokes; it would take their minds off the knowledge of Jerry's loss.

The trip to the car later was full of new learning for all of them. Because Jerry didn't know the layout of the house, the Bechtels needed to help. But how to help? Finally, Don and Donna each took an arm and, pushing, pulling, talking, and providing more help than Jerry needed, they proceeded out the door, down the porch and along a railing.

To those around him, Jerry seemed more quiet, thoughtful and subdued, but for Jerry there was no mental energy to waste. All his capacity was focused on the new sensations that rushed his consciousness. Where was the ground? Donna's hand was tight on his arm. . . . Gray – blindness was like being in a gray box. Out in midair, that was blindness too. Taking a step, but not seeing his foot touch the ground, not knowing what he was putting his foot on.

"OK, Jerry, we're at the steps. There are two of them."

Two steps. He felt a jolt as his foot hit hard on the step, farther down than he imagined.

"We're on the sidewalk, about six steps to the car."

The scuff of shoes was the next sound.

"One step down, over the curb, Jerry."

A latch clicked and a hinge squeaked as the car door opened.

"A little to the left, Jerry, and the seat will be right under you."

Jerry felt a hand on his head, pushing down and left. His shoe banged the door sill.

"OK, Jerry, you're in."

Yes, but what would they do at the church? Jerry thought. He usually had steps to climb, a box to mount to direct the orchestra. Precarious enough without being blind. Someone would have to lead him up and point him in the right direction. Someone would always be leading him. . . .

At the church, there was the normal discordant clatter of musicians tuning their instruments. Then, one after another, the students stopped, instruments in midair, as they watched the four people coming down the aisle. They seemed to be leading Jerry, lifting on his arms, watching every step he took, as if he were blind.

Blind! The members of the band were staggered. How could it be real? They were close to Franks, loved him as a friend and teacher. Many considered him the most giving, Christlike man they knew. If it could happen to him. . . . Heavy thoughts quieted them, as each tried to deal with it in his own way.

It was soon apparent, however, that the show would go on. Jerry, led to his place before the band, raised both arms, gave a downbeat and the smooth, full sound filled every corner of the sanctuary: "A Mighty Fortress Is Our God." Shining sound, shining like the golden reflection of the tubas and French horns on which Jerry fixed his eyes. The one sight left to him was light reflected off the horns.

The afternoon bus trip to Waukegan, Illinois, was

not the usual cacophony of 30 kids on respite from school. Instead of shouted insults and jokes, there were pockets of subdued talking, as if those assembled were attending a wake or returning home in the pre-dawn hours. Jerry, in the front seat of the bus, learned a new aspect of blindness. It took pleasure away from riding in a car or bus. Instead of the panorama of greening field and trees that usually unfolded before his eye on the world, Jerry saw gray. With nothing to attract his attention, sleep came easily, so he was quiet, and the kids, thinking not to discomfort him, did not make their usual cluster of draped, propped humanity around his seat.

Phil Landrum was a welcome respite from such awed silence. Phil, a childhood friend of Jerry's and a Wheaton, Illinois, writer-publisher of the *Christian School Magazine,* drove to Waukegan to hear the evening concert and take Jerry home with him for the couple of days between concerts.

When Landrum walked up the church aisle that evening there was the usual bleat and ascending notes of instruments warming up. At the end of one row a group of early arrivals stood watching, making occasional comments to one another, but Phil's gaze searched for his friend.

Jerry was sitting on a bench at the front. Because he was looking down, Landrum thought he might be working on music or going over notes; but when Jerry lifted his head and did not acknowledge Landrum's wave, Landrum studied the man he'd known since fifth grade. Franks had the demeanor of one listening. Instead of sideways movement of the head to accommodate the eyes, his head was tilted forward, and he leaned right or left to help him identify and assimilate the happenings around him. Landrum, assuming that Franks was suffering a recurrence of blindness, called out.

"Jerry!"

"Hey, Moose!"

And with that exchange of greetings they were back in the easy camaraderie of childhood, when Phil had been the one with the handicap and Jerry had watched out for him. When the two of them had learned that no one is abnormal, each person encounters situations that allow for growth not otherwise possible. Now it was Landrum's turn. Jerry's blindness was a hurdle they would work on together.

Jerry related what had happened.

"Are you seeing anything at all?" asked Phil.

"I could tell where to stand in front of the band because I could see light reflected off the tubas. But light is all I can see."

In the car on the way to Wheaton, Phil asked about Jerry's plans.

"We're gonna go on. If I quit, we'd have to cancel, and I'm not gonna cancel a 25-concert tour. I'll have Dottie come up to help me."

"When do you think she'll be here?"

"Well, my dad's in the hospital, you know. He's having open heart surgery. She'll leave as soon as she hears how he's doing."

At the Landrum home, Phil led Jerry through the one-story house, making him familiar with the floor plan.

"OK, Jerry, straight back from the living room are the kitchen and family room. If you go left out of the living room you'll find the bedrooms, and the room you'll stay in is on the left at the end of the hall. You're only five steps from the bathroom, OK?"

"OK." Jerry ran his hand along the wall till he came to the second door frame. "Hey, Moose, you aren't gonna watch the NCAA Championship tonight, are you?"

"You bet!" said Phil. "A man from Kentucky always watches Kentucky play."

"Hey, did you hear about the tornado that went through Kentucky?"

"No, what about it?"

"It did $50 million dollars worth of improvement." Jerry snickered.

"Better be nice to me, Jerry," said Phil, "I might lead you to a busy intersection and leave you there."

After Phil had made Jerry familiar with the placement of furniture and necessary items in the bedroom and bath, Jerry called Dottie.

"Dottie? This is Jerry."

"Hi, Honey."

"How's Dad doing?"

"Just fine. The surgery went well, and your mom's really relieved."

"Dottie, guess what?"

"What?"

"I'm blind."

"When did it happen?"

"When I woke up this morning I couldn't see."

"Is it like last Christmas?"

"No, it's both eyes this time. All I can make out is light and dark. I think you better have Rob bring you out here."

"OK, Honey."

The plans were made for Dottie's trip and then Jerry and the Landrum family settled into the visit as if it were any other time they'd been together. As always, Jerry exerted his unique sense of humor on all the members of the household. When Phil was working, even Charlie, a lethargic basset, was the object of Jerry's whimsy.

"Oh, Charlie, buck up! Don't sit there like a toad. You're better than that. It's not good self-image to think of yourself as a toad. You should think of yourself as a dog."

Dog, family, friends, all were treated to a constant barrage of corny jokes, quips and putdowns.

"Boy, Lois, you and Dottie are just alike. Bossy and hard to get along with. If you would go to the battlefield in Viet Nam the Viet Cong would surrender the minute you appeared. They'd take one look at you and the war would be over."

Twenty-five concerts in three states. The rich, full sound of a big band delighted audiences at every stop. With the brittle blare of trumpets, the mellow trombones, and French horns, and the beating rhythm of drums in "ride," the 30-member Dimensions in Brass moved from classic, to patriotic, to emotion-filled sacred, to Jerry's didoes of wit and whimsy.

About his anniversary: "We've been happily married for three years. Three out of 20 isn't bad."

About being blind: "Everybody asks me why I continue to drive my car, but you wouldn't ask me that if you'd ever ridden with my wife. . . . I do all the night driving because glare doesn't bother me."

About his work as consultant to instrument companies: "When I designed my first student model instrument and no one could afford to build it, they told me to design an instrument that could be built in this country for under $200.00. So I thought and thought, and what

I came up with was the funnel for $193.50."

With Dottie's help, most of the difficulties of mobility were overcome; but when Franks was performing he was alone on the podium. While he could see light, he positioned himself with the aid of the reflection off the horns; but when that little bit of sight was gone, a new way had to be devised so that he could find his place without Dottie helping every time.

The answer was a wooden box. One of his students, Loren Hoyt, made a box with sides two inches high in which Jerry stood while performing and directing. There was a bolt on the panel nearest the audience, so Jerry felt with his shoe and put his heel against it when directing, and his toe against it when playing a solo. It was nicknamed "the playpen."

Two weeks and 25 concerts in three states was a busy schedule, one that left little time for self-pity. But when sight did not return, in the quiet times after the troop of young people had dispersed to their host homes, Dottie and Jerry talked together, hoping and praying, and planning the steps they would take. They did not, at that time, envision the ways in which God had already answered Jerry's frantic "Lord, help!"

When Jerry arrived back in Winona Lake, Indiana, his family doctor sent him to a doctor in Kalamazoo, Michigan, who put a damper on any hopes he may have had about seeing again.

"You'd better be prepared to spend your life as a blind man. Your sight is gone."

Jerry listened quietly.

"Have you thought about what you're going to do for a living?"

"I'm going to do what I'm doing now," said Jerry.

"'Fraid not. There's no way you're going to be able to wave your arms and conduct. You're going to experience a tremendous amount of dizziness just from being blind. If you try to blow your horn or wave your arms, you could get so lightheaded that you'll fall off the stage.

"You know what you could do?" the doctor went on. "After blind school you could look into this special program in Washington, D.C., where blind people set up food stands. With your education and experience you could have your own stand in no time."

Jerry smiled at that. Even Doc Severinson had called

him "pudgy" on national television one evening. "I'd never make a dime," he said, "I'd eat up all the profits! And besides, I've already done 25 concerts and I didn't have any dizziness."

The doctor was silent. Jerry was wondering at what the doctor had said, ". . . so dizzy you'd fall off the stage." He hadn't experienced any of that. He'd gone on – only inconvenienced with getting his place on the podium. Well, God had promised it would be all right. Maybe that's what He meant.

Jerry visited five doctors after his return from the tour, and the final one gave him awareness of another way in which God had helped. A Pittsburgh doctor, he was one of only a few in the country who could do surgery through the temple, rather than through the cornea, to restore sight. Jerry's father accompanied him but was refused entrance to the examining room.

With a hand on the doctor's shoulder, Franks passed through the doorway to the examining room, leaving the murmur of voices and clamor of phones in the outer office. Silence eased his senses.

"There's a chair to your right, Jerry, a straight chair." The doctor's hand was on his arm, guiding. "Just a couple steps sideways. Now back. There you are."

"You've been blind how long now, Jerry?" An instrument rasped against a tray as the doctor picked it up.

"A couple of months now. Since Easter, March 26."

"I'm going to look into your eyes now, Jerry."

After the examination, Dr. Garrett pulled a chair close to Jerry and sat down.

"I'm sorry, Jerry, there's nothing I can do in the way of surgery, but we can examine you periodically for the next three years to see if conditions change." He ended with the lift of hope in his voice.

"Don't feel bad, Doc, that's what everyone else has said. But if I'm blind, I'm blind. I'm not going to worry about it."

"I'm encouraged to see that you have such a good attitude, Jerry. You'll be able to adjust better if you can accept it and go on." The doctor rose and walked behind his desk.

"There are a few things I usually tell my patients, and one of them is that with the loss of sight, you've lost 90 percent of your senses, so don't be reluctant to ask for help when you need it. Sighted people always like to help, but they don't know when or how to, so it helps put them at ease if you'll just say what you need when you need it.

"But," he went on, "don't make your wife your nurse. Try to avoid having her do everything for you. You'll both be better off."

"OK, Doc," Jerry answered.

"I think you'll be fine, Jerry. I wish more of my patients could be as accepting. Jerry, did you wonder why I didn't allow your father to come in here?"

"Yeah, a little."

"Well, I'm the last hope for many people, and when I say, 'I can't help you' they go crazy. I've even carpeted the walls because so many people react that way. Anyway, it's enough to deal with the patient in that situation, let alone their families. So that's why I don't allow anyone other than the patient in here."

"Anyone other than the patient." Jerry ran that over in his mind. Oh, yes there was! Jerry knew that God had entered that room with him, and was with him now, just as He had been all along. That was why he had escaped terrible trauma and hopelessness, and it was why he would be able to go on in a profession that he loved. Like he and Phil had decided a long time ago, there are all kinds of situations that people have to face and overcome; but God is always there to help.

Chapter 2

Music, "Moose" and Marriage

A summer morning, 1951, Uniontown, Pennsylvania.

The phone rang four times before Kitty Franks could get to it.

"Hello?" She turned away from the phone. "Boys, quiet down so I can hear." She spoke into the phone again, agitation in her voice. "Hello?"

"Hi," said Ruby Landrum. "How are you getting along over there?"

"Well, the boys are getting over the whooping cough, but I may be the next one in bed."

"Yes, I think I had the easy part. The three weeks they were with me they were too sick to cause much trouble."

"It's a shambles! Jerry is blowing his horn and Phil is marching in time to the music – on the sofa, to the chair and back to the sofa. I think the doctors who set six weeks as the quarantine period should have to take care of these two sixth-grade boys!"

Mrs. Landrum laughed. "Do you want me to come get my half of the inseparable duo? They should be able to get along without each other for a little while."

"No. Hard as it is to take care of them together, it's worse to take care of them apart. Jerry would be whining that there was nothing to do, or he'd be on the phone all the time.

"But you know something?" Mrs. Franks went on, grateful for a sympathetic ear. "Today I wish Jerry's father had never given him a mouthpiece when he was two years old."

Mrs. Landrum chuckled quietly. "But just think of what you would have missed. He wouldn't be playing solos in church all the time, and he wouldn't have played 'Praise the Lord and Pass the Ammunition' at a missionary meeting when he was four."

"Oh, so you've heard about that!"

"Yes, I've heard about it many times; the new minister's wife hears lots of things, particularly about a former minister's wife and her disapproval of things connected with the church."

"Well, it was really kind of touchy at the time, me being the organist and all, but I didn't think of the song as sacrilegious."

"I know you didn't mean any harm."

"I sure didn't. But today I might do harm!" She spoke more calmly. "I'm proud of Jerry – you know that. Most of the time I don't mind his practicing, but today I'd like to throw the horn in the river and watch it sink to the bottom. Or maybe I could do what he did when he was little and pack the plagued thing with modeling clay." She laughed. "That would put a stop to the noise."

"Well, I'm glad you still have your sense of humor; but if you want to get rid of Phil, just give me a call."

Music and a strong Christian home molded the young Jerry Franks. Christianity was lived and shared, along with the good-natured humor that bubbled up and spread over the landscape of their family.

The music was as available and natural as the air they breathed. His mother was an organist and pianist, and his father, the high school band director. When Jerry was two, his father gave him a trumpet mouthpiece. When Jerry learned to make a sound in it, his father attached an instrument, and when he was playing every song he heard "by ear," his dad decided he'd better be able to read notes. So he gave Jerry lessons. Soon the path was clear; music was the route and the goal. God was the guide.

Phil Landrum provided a shaping of Jerry Franks's character and understanding in a different way. Phil, Jerry's friend since fifth grade, had a problem. An affliction. Whispered, not spoken. Feared and misunderstood. Jerry Franks covered for him.

In 1951, once a week in Connellsville, Pennsylvania, the Child Evangelism Program was on the air:

"And now, with a duet, Jerry Franks and Phil Landrum of Uniontown."

Jerry and Phil stood before the mike. The pianist concluded her introduction and the boys started singing "What a Friend We Have in Jesus."

Jerry sang the alto, sometimes nudging Landrum's tones, at other times breaking free to a fifth progression. What fun to hear the harmony, to call up the proper note and find it there, leaping from thought to sound. Jerry loved to sing, melody or harmony, it didn't matter. A note was a note – fun!

As they started the second verse, Jerry felt a change in Phil. The arm beside his arm was no longer moving in easy rhythm, it was straight, rigid. And then Phil stopped singing.

Jerry looked out of the corner of his eye at his friend. Phil was gazing into space, staring without seeing. Jerry switched from an A to a C, Phil's note, and continued in the melody, singing what listeners took to be a solo. After about 30 seconds, Phil jerked, looked at the music and Jerry, listened a moment, and then picked up the soprano as Jerry sounded the alto again.

Phil's epileptic seizures were unpredictable, often leaving him in danger, as when he stopped in front of oncoming cars. Jerry, watchful and protective, pulled him out of danger, carried him home when a "grand mal" occurred on his paper route, and distracted teachers when Phil's episodes happened in class.

If Phil were reciting or reading and he suddenly stopped gazing glassy-eyed ahead of him, Jerry would send a book thudding or a pencil clattering to the floor. In the time it took for the teacher to look Jerry's way and make an apology to Phil for the interruption, Phil would be prepared to read again.

One warm fall day, however, when the Appalachian mountains around Uniontown were alive with color and the boys and girls were wishing themselves away from the confining classroom and the droning of reading students, Jerry got more than a look.

Phil was standing, reading from the assignment in the literature book, when he stopped in mid-sentence, his hands gripping the book. Jerry, in a seat near the window, studied Phil. Phil's hands were already tightening on the book. Staring and stiffening would be harder to disguise with Phil standing. Jerry looked for a means of distracting class attention.

Poised on the window sill to his left were the books of the student ahead of him. One quick swipe and they would hit the floor and wake everybody up. Jerry smiled to himself at the mental picture. Jerry leaned to his left, his eyes still to the front, and catching a corner of the stack, gave the books a push. The scraping of cardboard across gritty sill drew the owner's attention.

"Hey!" he said.

The class and teacher, as one, looked his way just in time to see a corner of the stack disappearing over the outer edge of the window sill. In the silence that followed, the books could be heard plop-plopping on the ground two stories below.

"Jerry Franks!" the scolding began.

But Jerry and "Moose" were friends. If one had a problem, the other helped. They shared an understanding that any affliction was just a hurdle to climb over. Phil had epilepsy – other people were skinny or fat. Phil had seizures, but it was still Phil inside that stiffening body. It was Phil who would emerge again, like a kid with a dirty face would still be the same kid when he came out from behind the dirt. Wasn't that how God saw people? Weren't Christians supposed to see the inside of people too?

Music, music, music. Jerry sang, played and practiced, becoming so proficient that his talent was soon recognized by those outside Uniontown.

In 1955, when Jerry was 17, his older brother, Dan, who played first flute with the Youngstown, Ohio, Philharmonic Orchestra, told Jerry that the orchestra would be having a concert that would include high school musicians. He thought Jerry should be included, so he had said to the leader, "Use my brother."

They did use his brother. Jerry played in the youth concert and then continued in several more concerts, driving five hours one way, and, when extra rehearsal was needed, often returning home at 4:00 a.m. and rising for school at 7:00 a.m.

Because he was a good student, however, his schoolwork did not suffer. Nor did it suffer when he missed

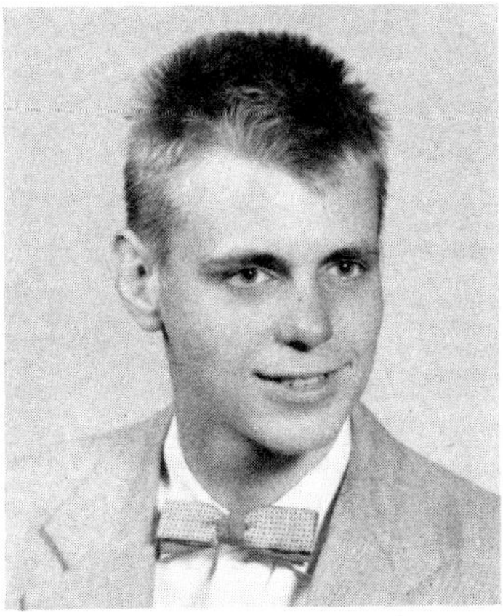

Jerry's high school graduation (1955)

school numerous times because of his playing taps for the funerals of VFW, American Legion and Am Vet members. When a funeral was scheduled, he was often picked up at school by a member of the organization, driven to the graveyard and then returned to the school. Sometimes, however, if the funeral was at the funeral home across from the high school, Jerry would cross the street and catch the "flower truck," a Cadillac, built much like a Chevrolet El Camino, that transported flowers from funeral to gravesite.

A diversion instituted by the youthful driver, and not altogether discouraged by fun-loving Jerry, was to drive up Summit Mountain and test the car to see how fast it would go. When they reached the top they would whiz down again, strewing flowers along the road for miles.

Woven into the pattern of his life from age 14 on was brown-haired, flashing-eyed Dottie Shaffer. They met at the Grace Brethren Church they both attended. Dottie looked over the boys at a church youth group meeting and decided that Jerry was the best they had to offer; Jerry looked over the girls and said to himself, "Well, all things considered, she's the best of the bunch."

They continued to think that way and settled into a long courtship that included the usual telephone calls at the dinner hour (a situation that Dottie's mother deplored), bus trips from his house to hers eight miles away, and the usual long walks and ice cream sundaes at the soda shop.

On one date Jerry and Dottie attended church and then went on to the soda shop. Afterwards, they dashed to the bus stop in a pouring rain so Dottie could catch a bus to her home. When Jerry took change out of his pocket to pay the bus fare, he looked at the coins in his hand and said, "That man at the soda shop gave me a nickel too much."

"Jerry, forget it," said Dottie. "We can give it to him the next time we go in."

But Jerry ran back to the shop through the rain to return the nickel. Dottie thought it was the stupidest thing she had ever heard of, but she admired his honesty.

Jerry's enrollment in college in 1956 didn't change his involvement with Dottie or his reliance on God and His laws as the guide for his life.

Music was the career goal. Music it had to be. But Grace College at Winona Lake, Indiana, his church college, did not have an instrumental program. So Jerry made a promise to God: he would go to another school, and if the Lord would guide him so he could get professional experience, he would teach in a Christian college so that other Christian young people could get professional training.

Dottie supported his decision; West Virginia University had what Jerry needed. So Jerry commuted daily to Morgantown, West Virginia, 25 miles south of Uniontown. This allowed him to be near Dottie and to continue the chauffeuring job he had held for a number of years.

He worked for three eccentric Jewish brothers, Harry, Julius and Samuel Schein. Harry and Julius were jewelers in Uniontown, and Samuel was an optometrist. Samuel was also a musician who knew Jerry's father. When the Schein brothers needed a chauffeur, Samuel decided that Jerry would be a good choice because they could talk music together.

Being a chauffeur for the Schein brothers provided quite a challenge to Jerry because Harry and Samuel had physical problems and all three brothers were nervous about cars.

Jerry learned to drive the big Buick Roadmaster so smoothly that even water wouldn't spill, because that is exactly what Harry had his feet in. Harry, who had an inflammation of the feet, needed to soak them as often as possible, and that included during travel.

Frail, fearful Dr. Samuel Schein, who always sat in the front seat, had asthma and kept his sprays and medicines in the glove compartment. Unfortunately, sitting in the front seat proved to be an aggravation to Samuel's asthma, because he watched the speedometer constantly, and any time it went over 50 miles per hour he would start gasping and rocking in his seat, saying, "Oh my! Oh my! Oh my!"

The car was meticulously cared for, the gas tank filled and the exterior washed after every use. One day, however, the car had only a quarter tank when they began the weekly drive to Pittsburgh. When the deficiency was discovered the "Oh my's" started.

"We're out of gas. Stop the car!"

"We still have a quarter of a tank, we don't need to stop," said Jerry.

From the back seat came: "If we're out of gas, my feet hurt. I can't walk."

"There's a house," said Julius. "Let's call a tow truck."

"We don't need to call a tow truck," said Jerry, "we're still running."

"If we don't stop, there might not be any more houses where we can call a tow truck."

"We have a fourth of a tank of gas, we don't need a tow."

"Oh my! Oh my! Oh my!" said Samuel.

The argument bounced back and forth for about 12 miles, until they came upon a gas station. In a chorus the brothers said, "Gas station, gas station! Stop, stop!"

"Where did that gas station come from?"

"It must be brand new."

"We're saved, God built a gas station!"

"Let's stop! Let's stop!"

Noises attendant to the car also upset the three brothers. One day when a light rain was falling and the wipers squeaked, the dialogue began.

"What's the matter with the wipers?"

"There's not enough water on the windshield," answered Jerry.

"Get them fixed."

"We don't need to; they pull on the glass and squeak when it's not raining very much, that's all."

"Oh my! Oh my! Oh my!" said Samuel.

"Get the car to a garage and get them fixed," said Julius.

Later, Jerry took the car to a garage.

"There's nothing wrong," said the mechanic, "they're just not wet enough."

"I know. Look at it anyway."

"But there's nothing to look at."

"I know. Look at it and send a bill."

"I'll just say I looked at it and tell them there's no charge."

"No, send a bill or they won't think you checked it."

Eccentric as the brothers were, they were even more generous. When Harry and Julius went to Pittsburgh to the jewelry outlets, they would often ask Jerry if he wanted to take anything to Dottie. So Dottie was the recipient of lovely things like jewelry boxes and gold-plated mirrors.

The purpose of one trip was a visit to a diamond cutter. As he was working on a stone, the cutter suddenly exclaimed, "This is the most perfect diamond I've ever seen."

"What a stone!" said Julius.

"Beautiful!" said Harry.

The brothers put it in a small envelope and took it with them. On the way home, they said to Jerry, "When are you getting engaged to Dottie?"

"I don't know. We've been going together six years. I guess we've always known we'll get married someday, but I don't know exactly when."

"You should have this diamond."

Jerry was stunned. "I couldn't afford such an expensive stone."

"We want you to have this."

"Thank you so much for offering, but I just couldn't manage it."

A year later, when Jerry decided to get a diamond for Dottie, he went to the Schein brothers jewelry store and said he was looking for a diamond engagement ring. The brothers brought a small, familiar envelope from the safe.

"We saved it for you," they said.

"I can't take it," said Jerry. "I can't afford it."

"You can drive it off; we want you to have it."

So Jerry "drove it off" and at Christmas in 1958 Dottie received a "perfect" diamond and a long-expected proposal.

June 13, 1959, was Jerry's and Dottie's wedding day.

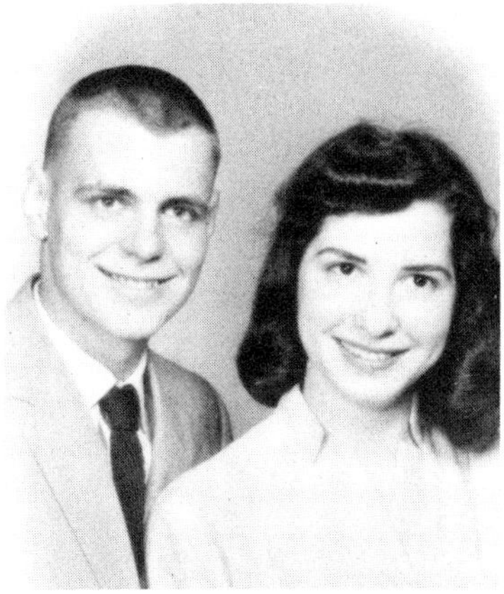

Jerry and fiancé,
Dottie Shaffer (1958)

A day so pure and clear that every tree on Summit Mountain, behind the Frankses' home, was a separate form of glistening green, shining back at the sun and directing attention to the simple cross at the peak. A perfect day for a wedding, or a ball game!

Jerry coached a group of kids in softball. They knew that Jerry wouldn't be available after his wedding, so they trooped up to his house to see if he and best man, Phil Landrum, could play one last time on the lot across the street from the Frankses' home. The game was on!

When his mother called, "Jerry, you have to get ready for the wedding!" he kept on playing. When Dottie called and wanted to talk to him, he yelled back to his mother, "Tell her to wait a minute. I'm up at bat!"

When the game was over, Jerry and Phil rushed to the house, got ready, and Jerry Franks married Dottie Shaffer the afternoon of June 13, 1959. He was 21; she was 20. Ahead lay two more years of school and experiences that prepared him as a nationally known trumpet player.

Chapter 3

A Decision

Fall 1959. The road to Morgantown.

Jerry's hands were tight on the steering wheel, his foot gentle but tense on the accelerator pedal, as his car moved slowly through the axle-high water.

He shouldn't have started across, but usually the gates across the bridge were closed when the water was too high for passage. If he could just keep the motor running, maybe he wouldn't regret taking the "back way" to school the morning after a heavy rain.

He knew the hazards that went with driving Road 857 the 28 miles to Morgantown each day: there were hills, hairpin curves and this lake that rose to cover the bridge after heavy rain. Still, Jerry considered it a better, quicker route because the large trucks that slowed traffic on 119 could not negotiate 857's inclines and curves.

Jerry breathed a sigh of relief as he guided the car onto dry pavement, through a sharp left turn, and up a steep hill. Maybe he would make the eight o'clock class after all.

Slants of sun flared through the trees, spotlighting a few gold leaves on fingertip branches, high above the graying mantle that had covered the forest floor. The day before, the golds, oranges, and reds had been a distraction to good driving, but overnight the pummeling of rain had changed the scene. It was sad to see the fall colors disappear in the mining areas of southern Pennsylvania and northern West Virginia. The rusty, dusty buildings and equipment seemed more dreary when the colors were gone.

As Jerry's car rounded a steep, sharp curve there was an opening in the trees, revealing the valley below and the towers and tipples of a coal mine. He'd known the shapes and sounds of coal-conveying tipples as they creaked and labored under the loads of coal they guided into trucks and rail cars. He knew the thunk, thunk of coal dropping into a truck bed because he'd accompanied his father on vacation and summertime runs to pick up and deliver coal. He'd watched the trains that ran on rails in the air and emptied their loads in the coke ovens.

Coal was West Virginia; West Virginia was coal, miles long and miles deep, and anyone who lived nearby knew its smell, sound and transportation. They also knew it as a source of income, even if only on a part-time basis.

The sights and surroundings were familiar, but like the forest around him, Jerry was entering a new season of his life: marriage, a wife, and a baby on the way. His schooling, his teaching, and working at his dad's store – Franks Musicland – were endeavors with new meaning.

Jerry thought of Dottie and their third floor apartment. It was interesting the way things worked out, the way the Lord worked things out. Who would have thought that he would be chauffeur to three eccentric brothers and thereby be able to have a beautiful diamond for Dottie? Who would have thought that they'd find a nice "starter" apartment because Jerry's dad rented a space in Mr. Pichinski's parking lot?

Very soon, though, they'd probably have to find another place to live. With the baby due in the spring, three flights of stairs might be too dangerous for Dottie. Maybe they could get into Lemonwood Acres, the new apartments built and subsidized by the government. The price was right, $25.00 a month. It would work out. The Lord would guide them.

Unlike Uniontown, which lay in a valley surrounded by mountains, Morgantown, West Virginia, scaled the hills. Like climbers "cramponed" to steep slopes, the houses, shops and schools, connected by ropes of road, clung to the forested hillsides. The university was no different. While students at other universities strolled rolling lawns, West Virginia University students climbed hills and mounted steps. But West Virginia was a good school and

Jerry was determined to absorb excellence in as many instruments as he could. Jerry parked his car, tucked his books more securely in the crook of his arm, hoisted his instrument and started climbing – 145 steps straight up! No wonder he was skinny.

The ride home was tense. A few extra minutes of practice, some slow traffic and he was running late. He had to be back in Uniontown by four o'clock to teach lessons and then help his dad until the store closed at nine. It all worked when he got away on time, but . . .

Then Jerry thought of the swollen lake and flooded bridge. Another delay if the water hadn't receded. Even without the flooding it was a dangerous area. A hill descended to a 90-degree turn and a narrow bridge. Drivers often misjudged the curve, and if they'd been drinking . . .

Jerry remembered an accident that had occurred on that turn. He'd been on his way home, braking as he descended the hill, when a car zoomed around him.

"Too fast!" Jerry had said aloud. "He'll never make the turn. What's the matter with that guy?"

Jerry's car had turned the curve at the very moment that the speeding automobile crashed through the open gate to the left of the bridge and went into the lake. The car was suspended on the water for a moment and then settled, nose down, leaving only the rear of the car above the surface.

Jerry stopped his car and dashed to the water's edge. Why didn't the guy get out? Maybe he was hurt. I can't swim, how can I help him?

"What happened?"

Jerry turned. A second car was parked at the edge of the road and a man was approaching.

"That guy must be crazy, he took the curve at about 50 and went right in the lake."

"Is he still in there?"

"Yeah. I can't swim, can you?"

"Yes, I'll get him. Why don't you see if you can find a phone and call for help?"

Jerry had sped to a house and called for an ambulance. The drunk driver had been pulled from his car and taken to the hospital.

Remembering the accident and what speed had accomplished, Jerry slowed and settled back against the seat.

Better to be late than never get there. He didn't want Dottie and the baby to lose out because he was too impatient to drive wisely.

Wisdom isn't always a dominant character of youth. Impatience and denial of mortality are. Jerry was no different. He rose early and retired late. He attended college, played "gigs" and when not playing "gigs," taught and worked in his father's store from 4:00 to 9:00 p.m. He skipped meals, grabbing cakes and candy, and then gorged late at night. His 120-pound frame fleshed out until he was overweight. And then in his mid-twenties, through an insurance physical, he met a family "friend": diabetes.

No big deal, that was Jerry's reaction. What was diabetes? His dad had it, his grandfather and aunts and uncles had it. They never had any trouble.

So Jerry took his orinase and continued his life full-speed ahead, a schedule that prohibited regular check-ups and worry about a faulty pancreas. When he finally got a check-up, he learned that the orinase had not been taking care of the insulin imbalance and that he needed insulin injections – the first in a series of changes that diabetes brought.

When Jerry was one year away from graduation, he was featured soloist at a Music Educators National Conference (MENC) at the University. MENC meetings featured orchestra and solo performances and educational seminars. A side benefit was the display of products having anything to do with music. Charles Colin, first trumpet for the DuMont TV network, soon to be the NBC orchestra, was present also, manning a booth displaying the wares of his fledgling publishing company. When Jerry walked by the booth, Colin called him over.

"Hey! Heard you play this morning. Not too bad."

"Thanks," said Jerry, noticing the badge pinned to Colin's jacket.

"I'm Charles Colin. I'd like to talk to you and hear you play again. Got a minute?"

"Sure," Jerry answered.

While Colin looked for an empty room, one of Jerry's classmates said, "Don't you know who that is?"

"Charles Colin, his badge said," answered Jerry.

"He's lead trumpet of the DuMont TV Network orchestra!"

"You're kidding! And he wants me to play for him!"

Later, after Colin had heard Jerry play, he said, "You're the best young trumpet player I've ever heard in my life."

"Thanks."

"In fact, you're better than I am, but if you say I said it, I'll deny it."

Jerry chuckled.

"I'm ready to give up full-time playing and go into full-time publishing and you're going to take my place. I'm going to get you a contract with the NBC orchestra in New York."

Jerry couldn't believe what he was hearing. Take his place! With the NBC orchestra! It was what he'd wanted to do all his life, since he was a little kid crying for his mom to find more band music on the radio.

"You go home," Colin continued, "and think about it over the weekend, and then we'll meet again on Monday."

The snowy mountain roads, the hills and curves, were inconsequential parts of Jerry's trip home. Close at hand, there for him to reach out and take, was a dream come true, a chance to be a pro, a chance for a decent living and a lifting of the financial burden from his father. Jerry was walking on air.

When he got home, Jerry shared his news with Dottie and then went to his father.

Mr. Franks looked at Jerry and said, "You're not quitting school."

"But . . ."

"It's a wonderful opportunity, I agree, but you need your education. And if you're good enough to do it now, you'll be good enough next year too."

Jerry looked at his father. Herb Franks wasn't just his father, he was his teacher, his music mentor. The man who'd given him that first mouthpiece and taught him how to use it. The man who'd guided him to learn to read music. Mr. Franks was wise in life and music, and Jerry respected his counsel. But how could he tell Colin?

When they met two days later in the West Virginia University music building, Colin was holding a telegram with authorization to offer Jerry a contract.

"Here it is, Jerry. We're leaving immediately to finalize the contract."

"I can't," was all Jerry could manage to say.

"When *could* you go?"

"I don't mean that." Jerry swallowed hard and went on. "I can't accept the offer."

"What? You must be crazy."

"No. I gotta finish school."

"Finish school? You don't need school!"

"My dad has worked hard and put me through this far, and he says I shouldn't quit."

"I don't believe it. You're crazy!"

Jerry's disappointment was so great that the shouting was an anticlimax. He could not react to Colin's invectives.

"I went to bat for you. Made arrangements. What am I gonna tell them? That Daddy said no?"

Jerry stood quietly, eyes cast down.

"Is that it? Is that your final decision?"

Jerry nodded.

"Well, here's your contract offer!" Colin ripped the pages before Jerry's face and let them fall to the floor. "Man, you'll never get off the ground with that kind of attitude!" He strode heavily out of the room.

The final year of school, that year that stood between Jerry and a good job, moved on lead feet. He knew he had to finish. He knew it would be better to have a degree, to get training in all the extra instruments. That had been his plan anyway. But bitterness over the lost opportunity made each day a chore, each 28-mile trip to Morgantown an aggravation to be endured. He wondered if he'd ever have such an opportunity again. Would Colin even speak to him?

After graduation, Jerry had a talk with Dean Richard Duncan, director of the music school at West Virginia University.

"Jerry, two things. I'm going to make you an offer and then give you some advice."

Jerry had asked for Duncan's advice; he listened attentively.

"First, I want you to know that you're the best trumpet player that has ever graduated in the 100-year history of this institution."

"Well, thanks."

"I'm going to offer you a job teaching trumpet here. We'll let you play and teach so you can get professional experience. That's my offer," Duncan continued. "Now, my advice is that you not take it."

"Yeah? Why?"

"Because what you need to do is get out and pursue your professional career. And when you get a teaching job, get a job in a grade school or junior high, and I'll hire you back at a lot more money because you'll really be worth something then."

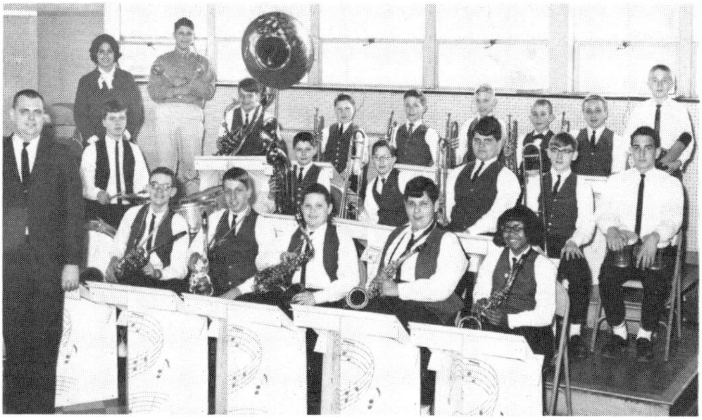

The Masontown Jr. High Stage Band (1963)

Jerry took Duncan's advice. He secured a position with the Albert Gallatin Schools, teaching fourth-to-ninth-grade music at Masontown Junior High. Then, because he didn't know how to get started with a professional career, he called Charles Colin.

"Hi, do you remember me?" said Jerry.

"Yes, I remember you," answered Colin.

"Well, I've graduated. It seemed to take a long time, but I guess it wasn't such a bad thing to finish school."

"No, it wasn't a bad thing," Colin agreed.

"Would you still be willing to help me?"

Colin helped Jerry get a contract with Buescher Instrument Company as soloist, doing demonstrations, clinics and public relations work. With the recognition acquired from that activity and his directing work with the Pennsylvania Band Masters Association, Jerry was soon being contacted to do studio work.

Studio work – back-up music for movies, recordings and commercials – required excellence and was a means to excellence. Because of the cost of musicians, time and production, and because composers often worked on music up to the time of recording sessions, Jerry and his fellow musicians had to be able to walk into a studio, look at the music and play.

The gathering of such talent in one studio was a means to learning for Jerry. Experienced in brass, knowledgeable in other instruments, and teaching all of them, the musicians gave the information Jerry sought in order to help the students he was teaching. One day, in a Chicago studio, Jerry asked a question of the Chicago Symphony's Fred Hemke.

"My junior high saxophone players can't play in the lower register. What do I do?"

"You're not teaching them clarinet embouchure, are you?"

"Yes, I am," answered Jerry. "That's what I was taught in college."

"They're not the same. A true saxophone embouchure requires more lower lip over the bottom teeth, which rounds the chin more and makes it more loose. It loosens the embouchure."

After four years of combining teaching, back-up and soloist-clinician work, two different kinds of offers came Jerry's way.

Dr. Herman Hoyt, Grace College president, was the featured speaker at the First Brethren Church in Uniontown in the spring of 1966. After the service, Dr. Hoyt, a very forthright man, spoke to Jerry.

"We want an instrumental program at Grace College and you're the man! Would you come for an interview?"

Jerry had never been to Grace College as an adult. The only contacts he'd had with it had been when the Grace College Choir performed in the Uniontown church or the public relations department showed slides of the campus.

"Sure I'll come for an interview," said Jerry.

Thus, with his accompanist, Nancy Hostetler, in tow, Jerry flew to Grace College and the Warsaw-Winona Lake area. He played a concert with the Warsaw High School band, and a solo at a Grace chapel service. He was interviewed and offered the job of "building an instrumental program at Grace."

Jerry liked the school. He felt that teaching at the college was a way of fulfilling his promise to the Lord and he saw the situation as a meshing of Grace's needs and his training. Grace needed an instrumental program, but could afford the salary of only one man; Jerry was one man who could teach all the instruments necessary for the formation of a band or orchestra. He said yes.

Two weeks later came a second offer and a real testing of Jerry's resolve.

Jerry appeared at a Pennsylvania Bandmasters Association meeting as a soloist and guest conductor with the U.S. Marine Band. In the audience was Ray Brown, father of Les Brown. After the concert, Mr. Brown approached Jerry and said that he thought Jerry should consider working with the Les Brown Orchestra. Not only did he speak to Jerry, he spoke to his son, and when Jerry returned to his hotel room, Les Brown called and asked Jerry if he would audition.

Then, just hours later, Jerry was approached about a job as soloist and assistant conductor with the U.S. Marine Band.

Jerry knew the opportunities being offered to him. The Les Brown Orchestra, soon to appear on "The Hollywood Palace," was featured on the "Dean Martin Show," and a regular with Bob Hope on his trips to service installations around the world; the Marine Band job promised the extra benefit of Jerry becoming conductor when the acting conductor stepped down. It was time for heavy thinking.

Les Brown, Bob Hope, Dean Martin. All this at his fingertips, and he was going to Grace College, where there was no active musical program, no students to teach. But he'd made a promise, and he knew that the Lord opened doors to help Christians keep their promises, so if the Lord was guiding him to Grace, that's where he would go. Jerry looked westward.

Chapter 4

I Promised the Lord

September 1966, Winona Lake, Indiana.

In 1966 Winona Lake was a quiet adjunct to its larger neighbor, Warsaw. But when it was established in 1895 as a "vacation spot with a religious environment" it was "where the action was".

Planned with the assistance of Dwight L. Moody and Bishop John H. Vincent, and developed by the financial support of John M. Studebaker, H. J. Heinz, Alexander McDonald and R. G. LeTourneau, it was guided by a forward-thinking board of directors. They established a trolley line between Warsaw and Winona Lake and a highspeed electric railroad to Goshen, Peru and intervening towns and townships.

In order to power these trains, the directors conceived and built a powerhouse that not only propelled the trains, but provided power for the Winona Utility and Heating System. Then, exhibiting true economy and ecological wisdom, they decided that the exhaust steam from the powerhouse could be conserved and used to heat the hotel, school building, greenhouse and 50 private homes!

No grass grew under the feet of these early founders, nor did it grow when thousands of visitors trod the shaded lawns and quiet beaches to attend concerts, operettas or Christian conferences.

When Jerry trod the streets of Winona Lake in 1966, he saw numerous memorials to the people who had made

Winona Lake a nationally known gathering place. He could see the Billy Sunday Tabernacle, with its rough, wooden benches and sawdust floor, where musicians Galli-Curci, Schumann-Heink, Swarthout, Zimbalist and Sousa performed, and where William Jennings Bryan spoke and Billy Sunday roared.

He could walk where James Whitcomb Riley and Theodore Drieser had walked, and visit the stone house perched on the side of the hill where Sunday had lived. He saw the wide porches of the Winona Hotel, where thousands had walked or rocked during their sabbaticals to the non-denominational Winona Lake Bible Conferences.

He was in a place where there had been great creativity and energy, and he would need just that if he were to establish a new endeavor at Grace College. For, when Jerry had surveyed the department he was to head, he'd found that there was virtually no department at all. Richard Messner, who had other responsibilities, had been guiding what musicians there were, but for the most part, there was no instrumental music program, no music stands, no music, no instruments and no rehearsal hall.

After some discouraging moments and thoughts about what might have been, Jerry sat in his office at Byer Hall, a large house on the corner of Kings Highway and Pierceton Road, and studied the situation.

Grace College, 12 years old, had none of the musty, ivy-covered edifices of older institutions. Its buildings, McClain and Alpha Halls, the main classroom building, Seminary Building and gym, were low, made of red brick with white facings and laid among pleasant, green slopes and drives. The buildings exhibited the philosophy of its founders: adequate, comfortable, for the singular purpose of educating Christian young people.

But there was no place to rehearse a large band. Byer was an older home on the west edge of campus. The rooms were office size, not rehearsal-hall size. Where would he put a band?

But wait a minute, Jerry said to himself. In order to need a rehearsal hall, you have to have a band, and you don't have one. Better find musicians first. Jerry decided to visit Bill Snap.

Bill Snap, a fine clarinetist, and his wife, Emily, a flutist, owned a music store. Lame and helpless when it came to walking, Snap let his music do the frolicking for him. Snap had organized a summer band that played at Center Lake Park in Warsaw, but a lack of funds had curtailed the number of performances.

Jerry suggested that they pool their assets. With Snap's people and Jerry's department budget, a concert band might be created after all. Grace College officials supported the idea, so Jerry and Bill struck a bargain. Jerry would provide the music and whatever students he could find, and Snap would recruit community musicians.

Recruiting instrumentalists at Grace College turned out to be as popular as finding volunteers for Viet Nam. Jerry walked the halls of Grace College buildings, collaring students on their way to and from classes. He talked with kids in the dorm lounges and stopped them on campus. The reasons varied, but most of the time the answer was no.

"I played in high school, but I don't have time now."

"I can't play an instrument."

"Me? Are you kidding?"

One student said it in another way: "I played in high school and it was a great band, so there's no way I'd play in your rot-gut outfit!"

At the end of the recruitment, the score was Franks – 7; Snap – 45. An inauspicious beginning, but a beginning. They looked to the next step, a place to rehearse.

The Westminster Hotel, a huge, old building with large dining rooms to the back right and left of the lobby, had housed every kind of visitor to the Winona Lake area. It was now going to house an orchestra. Jerry secured the Rainbow Room, the dining room on the left of the lobby.

But the Rainbow Room was a popular place for holiday parties, and by the time the college/community band had been organized, it was Thanksgiving time. So, every Wednesday at 4:00 p.m. Jerry had to call the hotel to see if a dinner was scheduled. If there was, he then called all 52 members of the orchestra and cancelled the 7:00 p.m. rehearsal. Franks may have left West Virginia behind, but he was still finding a lot of mountains to climb!

Funds were limited, and the college had no experience with bands and rehearsal halls, so administration officials were in a quandary as to where the concert band could rehearse. But Jerry was committed to an instrumental program. If all they needed was a rehearsal hall, he'd find one.

Jerry rented the band room in the Warsaw Junior High building on Main Street in Warsaw. After two weeks of practice, however, rehearsals moved again; the Winona Lake Christian assembly had donated the use of the Rodeheaver Auditorium. Thus, every Wednesday for the rest of the school year, Jerry, using a pick-up truck from Grace, transported instruments, music and stands to the stage of the auditorium, where the orchestra practiced and prepared for a concert in the spring. The concert established the Grace College/Community Concert Band as a viable, positive part of the community.

During the 1966-67 school year, Jerry had done more than practice with the band on Wednesday evenings. He continued his soloist-clinician work with Buescher, his back-up work in cities like Chicago, New York and San Francisco, and he taught lessons to his first – and only – student, Bob Stone, a transfer from Bob Jones University.

Most of the time during Bob's senior year, Bob had Jerry's full attention, not just during private lessons, but also in percussion, brass pedagogy and woodwinds classes. Stone and Franks practically "lived together" in the classroom, the orchestra and even on trips to hear other artists. Stone remembers a trip to Elmhurst High School at Fort Wayne to attend a jazz clinic presented by Doc Severinson. After the clinic Jerry and Bob went to the stage to see Doc, whom Jerry had known when he was doing studio work in New York. Jerry picked up Doc's horn from the piano and said:

"Hey, Doc, what's this? A Getzen? That's like saying 'skunk.' " Jerry chuckled.

"Hey – Jerry, how you doing?" said Doc.

"Great. How'd you come to play a Getzen?"

"Well, they've come out with a brand new model, and I've signed on with them."

And the two were off on their favorite subject – horns, music, and playing – while Jerry's student listened in awestruck silence.

Later, over lunch, Bob took courage and asked Doc a question: "I'd like to be a studio musician. How would I get started?"

Doc was not encouraging. "I've spent eight hours a

day for years playing and traveling, and I'm only one in a million who've made it. The odds are really against you . . . and besides, I've paid a high price for it, in how it affects my family."

In the course of their time with Doc, Jerry asked Bob to notice Doc's teeth, which came to a point in front and had a slight separation. Jerry felt that Doc had the ideal mouth for a trumpet player because air could get through and the forward wedge in his teeth prevented the horn from cutting off circulation to the lips.

Doc disagreed. He thought the emphasis was on breathing and practice. "If a good player practices six hours a day, you practice eight hours a day to be better than he is."

Bob was not to learn the wisdom of Jerry's theories about teeth until much later, but he did have cause to realize the value of Jerry's skills and input when it came time to do his student teaching.

Bob Stone was one of the first students from Grace College to do his student teaching in the Warsaw Community Schools. He was "on the spot" because he was one of the first, a representative of Grace, and because he would be doing his practice teaching under Bazil O'Reilly, a director highly esteemed by Indiana music educators.

Jerry made the arrangements and gave Bob a most important gift: encouragement and confidence. Bob felt that Jerry, who continually reinforced him with "You can do it, you won't have any problems," did more to build his confidence than any other person.

Bob's time with O'Reilly was a success. O'Reilly wrote a letter to Grace congratulating them on "the best student teacher I've had in my history of teaching."

Bob's success was only the tip of the effect that Jerry's teaching was to have on a succession of students. In September of 1967, because of recruiting in Grace Brethren churches the previous year, Jerry had a musical instrument department of 11 students and he was looking for a way to use them – something that hadn't been done before.

With Jerry's love for band music, it was natural that his thoughts went that way. A brass group, he thought, a brass group that played sacred music! That would be great! Then Jerry prayed, dedicating the new group to the Lord, and praying that it would be unique, a special witness for those who heard it.

As the year proceeded, the "Grace College Brass Choir" traveled with the vocal choir, recruiting potential students for the college as they went. They were also trying to think of a better name for the group. Finally, in a quiet moment, Jerry found the name: "Dimensions in Brass."

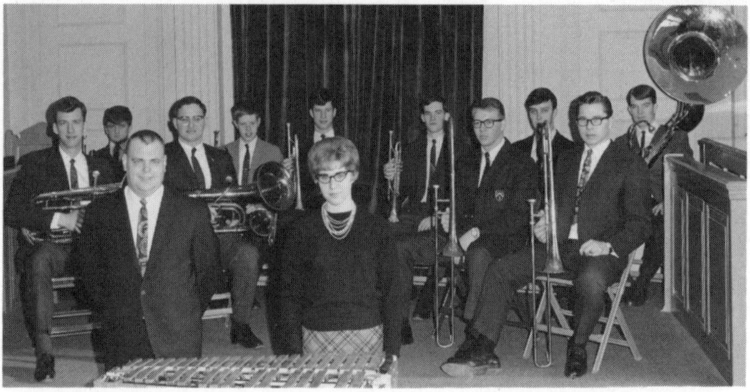

The original Dimensions in Brass of Grace College (1967)

Dimensions was a name and a description of the group in ensuing years. For it grew in numbers, spread its sphere of awareness and influence and achieved levels of performance that left Jerry little time to worry about where he would find a department.

His main worry was where to put the Dimensions in Brass for rehearsals. In their North Hall quarters they outgrew the living room so that other areas had to be pressed into use. The main brass part was in the living room, the bass were in the foyer and the drums on the front porch, while Jerry shouted from the dining room: "OK, now, the tempo goes like this."

When President Hoyt visited one day and saw Don Bechtel practicing his horn in a bathroom, he asked, "Isn't that a bathroom?"

"Yes," answered Jerry.

"Why is he in there?"

"Because we have too many students; they practice where they can."

Within three weeks Jerry was notified that he would be moving to East Hall.

From traveling with the Grace Choir as back-up, the Dimensions in Brass grew and progressed until it was traveling alone, a second musical ambassador from Grace College. And as a result of playing at Grace College ball games, the Dimensions developed a "pop" program that was in demand by public schools and civic groups.

In the early '70s Otis Bowen was the featured speaker at one of these gatherings in the Warsaw High School Auditorium. Bowen thought that Jerry was the best triple tonguer he'd ever heard, a qualified endorsement since Bowen had played a trumpet himself in high school.

Thus, when it was Indiana's turn to host a governors' conference, Bowen suggested that the planning committee include the Dimensions in Brass on the program. To Bowen, Jerry Franks reflected credit on Indiana and represented what was exemplary in people in general: excellence in his craft, inventiveness, conscientiousness, determination, and a positive impact on young people – qualities he enumerated in a citation presented to Jerry after his performance in June of 1979.

As Director of Instrumental Music and Artist-in-Residence at Grace College, Jerry was able to continue a schedule he started when teaching at Masontown Junior High. He taught classes and private lessons and directed the band, but when there was clinician work, he traveled.

The horn he demonstrated at that time was a Conn. Because Selmer had bought Beuscher and Jerry was not satisfied with the instrument he was given, he was open to a proposal made by Conn Instrument Company of Elkhart, Indiana.

"Jerry, this is Brooks Dawson of Conn Instrument Company."

"Oh, yeah, how are you?"

"Great, Jerry. Listen, I'm assistant advertising manager and I've been authorized to call you. We have a horn we think you might like."

"What is it?"

"A Conn 60B. If you like it, we'd like to have you work for us. Want to try it?"

"Sure. I'll try it."

Jerry went to Elkhart, liked the horn and said yes to a contract, which started a long association with Conn and Dan Hencken, owner of Conn and 21 other music and instrument companies.

Hencken, who had been a professional musician, was

delighted to have Jerry as a clinician. From his long years as a musician and participant at band and orchestra conventions, he knew that Jerry was one of the finest trumpet players and brasswind instructors in the country and could have had his choice of music companies.

Keeping "the finest" musicians was essential to Conn and other instrument companies. A clinician had to be able to play well in order to make the instrument look good when he appeared as guest soloist and director with various bands around the country. He also had to exhibit an excellence that would engender the respect of other musicians. He had to be a good speaker and teacher so he could help students with breath control and embouchure development, and he had to be able to tell high school, college and professional conductors how to improve *all* brasswind sections.

In addition, a clinician was expected to help in the development or revision of instruments. Thus, whenever Conn brought out a new model it was sent to Jerry for testing, suggestions or approval.

Because Jerry wanted to be able to be more specific than to say, "I like it," or "I don't like the way this horn blows," he decided to learn more about horns. Soon he was visiting the plant, peeking over shoulders and asking questions of engineers, plant managers and acousticians about venturis, bell stems and lead pipes. Jerry was prepared when Conn called about a new venture.

"Jerry, why don't you help us design a new horn?"

"Sure," answered Jerry. "Sounds interesting."

"We have plans to do a new student model cornet and we were thinking it would be great if a trumpet player, someone who actually plays a horn, would design it, instead of someone with a slide rule."

"A cornet, you say?"

"A cornet and a trumpet actually. How about it?"

"Sure. It would be a great challenge."

To sell the new horn, the Conn Director's Model for students, Juhl Advertising of Elkhart, Indiana, devised a plan whereby Jerry traveled to Chicago, Los Angeles, Dallas, New York and San Francisco and gave concerts on horns taken off local dealers' shelves and handed to him directly before he played. The plan worked. The Conn Director Model became Conn Instrument's most popular model up to that time.

In his capacity as soloist, Jerry often performed as guest soloist for high school and college bands. Often these trips had interesting side benefits.

Soon after the 1967 recording of "Trumpet Conversations," Jerry's first solo album – done through Brethren Missionary Herald Company – Jerry was flown to Los Angeles, California, to perform for a BMH bookstore opening. In the course of this tour, the pastor of one of the churches where he played contacted Dodger Stadium and suggested that Jerry might be a possible performer for pre-game shows and the national anthem. As a result, Jerry was invited to speak with Red Paterson, vice president of the Dodgers, and ultimately to play at Dodger Stadium. He was given an open invitation to play there whenever he was in town and did so upon several occasions.

During a 1977 trip to San Diego, where he gave two concerts and a clinic at Point Loma College, Jerry's student driver picked him up after a rehearsal and said, "I hear you like cars."

"Yeah, that's right," answered Jerry.

"You wouldn't believe the limousine that Jackie Gleason's got!"

"Yeah, where'd you see it?"

"At the resort where I'm doorman; Gleason's staying there."

"What's it like?"

"It's a new 1978 Lincoln limo. It's a gorgeous car! I know the chauffeur and I know where the limo's parked – down at the Fox Theater where Jackie Gleason is rehearsing. Would you like to look at it?"

"Man! Yeah! Let's go!"

Outside the Fox Theater sat the three-tone cordovan limo, long, sleek and imposing, taking up more than its share of space along the curb.

"Man, oh, man, would you look at that!" said Jerry.

"I'll go in and get the chauffeur," said Jerry's driver, as he stepped out of the car.

When Jerry's driver and Gleason's chauffeur came out of the theater, the chauffeur unlocked the limo and invited Jerry in. Jerry settled onto the plush seat and studied the interior.

"Would you look at that!" he exclaimed, "A TV, bar, refrigerator and telephone!"

"Isn't it something?"

While they were talking, Gleason's chauffeur, who had been informed by Jerry's driver that Jerry was a performer, went into the theater and told Gleason that there was a trumpet player outside who was admiring his car. A proud owner, Gleason went outside to show off the car himself. He crawled in with Jerry and described all the special features to Jerry.

As they were talking, a crowd, anxious to see Gleason, assembled outside the car. Because of the crush of people outside the theater, Professor Erwin Corey, who shared the bill with Gleason, was unable to get to the theater and decided to join the occupants of the car.

"Wow! I never saw such a car," said Jerry.

"Probably not," said Gleason. "We added four inches on the bumper to make it the longest limo ever built. I call it 'The Great One.' "

They shared a laugh and then Jerry said, "And with this phone you can call any place in the country?"

"Yeah. Hey, let's call your wife back in Indiana. She won't believe that you're sitting in the back of my car."

As they talked, exchanged tickets to performances, and shared the special conversation of car enthusiasts, the crowd watched outside.

In addition to Jerry's traveling as soloist, guest conductor and recruiter for Grace College, and because of it, greater numbers of young instrumentalists were attending Grace. Jerry taught all of them in the classroom or in private lessons. Soon students were added to those numbers from high schools and colleges in Ohio, Michigan and Indiana. College students came from Indiana University, the University of Michigan, Bethel, Marion, Manchester, Taylor, Ball State University and Indiana State University. In the summertime students came from as far away as the University of Texas and San Francisco. At one time, a total of 90 students were under Jerry's tutelage.

It wasn't long before Jerry was being recognized in the *International Who's Who in Music, Who's Who in Percussion* (a recognition that Jerry particularly cherished since he was not a percussion specialist), and the *Outstanding Educators of America.* But his most prized recognition was being asked to solo at the Midwest National Band Clinic.

The Midwest National Band Clinic was a convention for band directors at all levels, junior high, high school, college, military and professional. Though called "Midwest" and "National," it was *international* in scope and provided a meeting place for all the components of music-making: the director-teachers and their students; the specially chosen bands that provided back-up for the best soloists; the publishers who displayed their music; the instrument companies that exhibited horns; and even the vendors who sought contracts with directors for annual fund-raisers.

Every December, in a large meeting room of Chicago's Palmer House Hotel, signs, booths and banners announced "Conn, Selmer, DeFord, Volkwein, Fischer, Sausages, Cheese, Light Bulbs" and "The Finest Chocolates for Your Fund-raiser."

Music publishers outlined the shape of their booths with their latest compositions and arrangements and large signs that said: "Hear the Million Dollar Band Play this Volkwein arrangement at 2:00 p.m. in the ballroom!" Highly polished instruments reflected the overhead lights and the distorted figures of strolling instrumentalists – their shirts open and hats askew – as they juggled instruments and nibbles of sausage, cheese, nuts and "The World's Finest Chocolates." Above the call of vendors, buzz of voices and shuffle of feet, there was the occasional "squark" of a clarinet or blaring scales of a trumpet warming up in adjacent rooms.

To Conn owner, Dan Hencken, the Midwest National Band Clinic was a "never miss" occasion. It was where the best and the most in band music assembled and he wanted to be there, to show his instruments and to meet directors, teachers, and professional band leaders. Also, he attended because some of the best soloists in the world performed at the Clinic and he could make contacts, discussing amid the exciting hurly-burly the possibility of their representing Conn Instrument Company.

The hurly-burly would have been attractive enough, however, for Hencken, like all musicians in love with band music, liked to absorb everything that was bands, music and a convention for band music.

To Jerry, one of the Conn soloists that Hencken exulted in hearing, going to the Midwest National Band Clinic was a chance to meet instrument people from all over the world. He could see what was new in instruments, swap tips with other directors and play with the "best".

Jerry was invited to play with the "best" three times at the Clinic. One year, he played with Harold Backman's Million Dollar Band, an all-pro band made up of musicians from the U.S. and foreign countries. Another year he played with the Merl Evans All Circus Band, and a third time he was a soloist.

To Jerry, it was the "Oscar" for band musicians, musicians honoring the best of their peers, and he was delighted to be honored. But he was also delighted just to be there, soak up the sound, smell, sight, touch and taste of horns and bands. To hear the tootle of flute, blare of horns and thump of drum – sounds that had thrilled him since he was four, and had motivated his career choice.

And his career choice was to teach Christian young people, the occupation in which his brilliance manifested itself.

Chapter 5

"Like Abdul-Jabar's Skyhook"

A morning in the mid '70s. Jerry's office in East Hall.

Jerry drew a large oval on the board and pointed at it. "Now, this is you. It might not have your big blue eyes, but it's you."

He drew a group of circles around the base of the oval. "These are your abdominal muscles, see?"

He drew a line across the top of the oval. "If you breathe above this line," he put a hand on his upper chest and inhaled, "you're using the weakest part of your breathing apparatus. If you take a deep breath and use the abdominal muscles, you have all kinds of breath and control."

By the mid '70s, hundreds of students had heard Jerry's descriptions of the diaphragm and its workings, and thousands more had heard it from those hundreds.

Henry Adams once wrote that "a teacher affects eternity; he can never tell where his influence will stop." That is true of Jerry Franks. Like the branches of a tree spreading its shadow wider with each year's growth, or the roots of that tree sending out shoots from which new roots grew, Jerry's teaching reached into the music world.

His students became music teachers and band directors, and their students became music teachers and band directors. People like Don Bechtel, director of Cuyahoga Valley Christian Academy of Akron, Ohio, whose group was the only band from a Christian school to win at State Music Contest. People like Bob Stone, who in the three years he was there, built a band program from 40 to 300 students at Norwell High School near Fort Wayne and won repeated State Fair championships. Bob's students, Joe Moore, trumpet with the Marine band and Larry Whittenberger, trombone with a studio band, were living demonstrations of Jerry's teaching ability through Bob's teaching ability. People like Mark Van Cleave, lead player with the Buddy Rich Orchestra, who went on to be director of the Shrine Circus Band.

Jerry's students moved out into the music world, appearing with the South Bend, Fort Wayne, Chicago, Cincinnati and NBC symphony orchestras; with the Boston Pops, military bands, and with Christian groups such as "Truth" and Bill Gaither.

His music management students also had impact: Denny Leistner, later to do sound reinforcement for the Gaithers and for the opening and closing ceremonies of the 1987 Pan Am Games; Kevin Crawford, vice president of Reider Printing Company in Anderson, Indiana; Dave Stroup, with Selmer-Ludwig; and Dave Melton of Lexicon.

Wherever they went, his students carried their excellence and word of what Jerry had done for them, and they cited Jerry's 14 playing skills and his teaching ability as the reason for their success:

"He is unequaled in his teaching techniques; he understands how to make the sound and he tells us how to do it."

"He can bring a band of mediocre players up to par faster than anyone I know."

"He teaches you how to play so you can play any song put in front of you. You don't have to concentrate on different things, just play."

"He builds confidence; by the time he gets done, you believe you can handle the job."

"He can teach how to teach others – absolutely essential when you're right out of college and you have to be able to teach kids so they get it fast and don't get discouraged. Using what he taught me in music theory, I taught theory to my kids, and those that went to I.U. all tested out in theory."

"I don't think Jerry realizes how important his teaching is."

Jerry, the root carrying mental nourishment to the small shoots, is a teacher in the truest sense. Constantly asking questions, observing, examining and evaluating, he owes much of his learning to his youngest students. Fifth graders were not reluctant to ask questions when they didn't understand. "How do you get that sound? How do you play so low? How do you move your fingers so fast? How do you do that?"

"How do you do that?" they asked again and again, and more often than he liked, Jerry had to say, "I don't know, but I'll find out."

He was teaching as he'd been taught: explaining and demonstrating. But it was one thing to explain and demonstrate, and another entirely to help students understand how to use the horn, how to make a sound. So he studied himself and others.

How were his chin and mouth shaped when he blew? What did his diaphragm do when he hit a high note? What portion of the muscles was he using? How could he keep kids from pressing the horn too tightly against the mouth? What would help kids with half-valve slurring?

And since so many singular skills were necessary in playing a brass instrument, how could they possibly learn them by sitting in a band playing notes? That was starting with the end product and working backwards. Like putting Kareem Abdul-Jabar in a game before he knew how to shoot a skyhook.

How did Adbul-Jabar learn enough to go into a game? Jerry asked himself. Abdul-Jabar probably bounced a ball in the backyard over and over. Then he shot at the basket over and over and over. He got the moves down pat: fake, step away, turn and shoot. By the time he got into a game with five guys on him, he didn't have to think, "How do I shoot a skyhook?" He let reflex action take over. Fake, step away, turn and shoot. Two points! That's what musicians needed. They needed to know the skills before they got in the game.

Lots of teachers were teaching, but their students didn't always know how to play. Maybe teachers didn't really know how they achieved a sound. A lot of pros didn't either. They said they did it one way because that was the way they were taught. But in the process of working toward better tone, higher notes or greater endurance, they had developed their own methods and hadn't analyzed how they did it.

Analysis seemed to be the answer, then informing the student how the instrument worked, how he must function physically to operate it, and then encouraging him to practice until it was a reflex action.

So where would he start? How would he take students from *Dick and Jane* to *War and Peace* and still preserve their love of the activity? How could he prepare college students to be effective teachers? Well, he'd just start at the beginning, with the introduction to the horn, analyze how he played and then tell the kids how they could do it.

What resulted were the 14 playing skills that were to be so helpful to Jerry's students:

SOUND

In order to get a good sound on a brass instrument, open the teeth, correct overbites by pushing the lower jaw forward, and place the back of the tongue in the "Ah" position in order to open the throat.

PIVOT FOR THE LOW REGISTER

In order to get into the low register, the oral cavity must be made larger to depressurize the air. This is done by dropping the lower jaw and the back of the tongue and changing the temperature of the air stream from cold to warm.

FINGERS AND SLIDE

To play cleanly, valves must be slammed very hard with the fingers and the slide must be snapped by the wrist into each position, being smoothly controlled at the same time by the use of the forearm.

SINGLE TONGUE

Place the tip of the tongue behind the top teeth in the general area of where the teeth and gums come together; establish a vertical motion with the tongue as opposed to a horizontal one; use the syllable "da" to articulate; avoid tonguing between the teeth; concentrate on the fact that it is the force of the air hitting the lips that causes the attack and that the tongue does not tongue, but is merely a valve that releases the air – all important to single tonguing.

TRIPLE TONGUE

Develop the back of the tongue using the syllable "ga" before attempting the triple tongue. The tip of the tongue can be used to help develop the back of the tongue by comparing one to the other in speed and sound of attack.

When using the syllables "da da ga", in order to triple tongue, it is important that the "ga" not be inserted in the middle as in "da ga da" but kept on the end, "da da ga". Many teachers and books advocate the use of "ta ta ka" for the tongue syllables. These are not practical syllables for speed and lightness, and the only way to increase speed is to bring the tip and back of the tongue closer together, decreasing the motions of the tongue. This is done by moving the tip of the tongue higher in the mouth and the back of the tongue more forward in the mouth. This will automatically result in the use of the "da da ga" syllables, even though the player may be unaware of such a change.

DOUBLE TONGUE

After triple tonguing has been accomplished, double tonguing is an easy sidestep. Use the syllables "da ga" and the transition from triple to double is easy. Saying the syllables for both double and triple tonguing speeds the process of learning multiple tonguing.

BREATHING

Brass instruments are called wind instruments because air is the fuel. The breathing mechanism not only provides the fuel but also is the source of air pressure that is used to control the instrument. The air pressure must remain constant at all times. The pressure is created by tightening and lifting of the abdominal muscles and the control and regulation of the air pressure is accomplished in the oral cavity. This is done mainly by the positioning of the back of the tongue through the use of syllables and by the use of the pivot for the low register and the pivot for the altissimo register.

VIBRATO

Different styles of music lend themselves best to a particular vibrato: hand, slide, lip, jaw, and diaphragmatic vibrato. It is good for a player to learn several types of vibrato and employ them where they best suit the style, rather than making one type fit all.

WARM UP

Warm up to stimulate blood flow to the lips and to relax muscles in the embouchure. The best way to accomplish this is by playing low and slow for a prescribed amount of time which will vary with each player and his requirements of performance. The longer and more demanding the practice or performance period, the more vital the warm-up becomes. Warming down is also a good practice to follow, especially after heavy playing, and involves the same principles as warming up.

FLEXIBILITY

The best way to develop flexibility (the ability to make rapid and accurate breath pressure changes) is through the use of lip slurs and lip trills, which are not done with the lip, but are accomplished with the back of the tongue. The back of the tongue regulates the air pressure through the use of syllables: "ah" in the low register, "ooh" in the middle and "ee" in the high register.

Flexibility is very important, not only for register changes, but for controlled playing within a register. Lip slurs and lip trills are used to develop the rapid and accurate manipulation of the back of the tongue for the purpose of gaining flexibility, not for the purpose of merely being able to lip slur and lip trill.

HIGH RANGE

The shape of the teeth is a major factor in a person's ability to play high on a brass instrument. He must have what we call a "pressure point" on the upper and lower teeth in order to perform in the altissimo register. Without a pressure point, pressure is focused on the lips near the corners of the mouth – where the lips are not inside the mouthpiece – cutting off the blood flow to the vibrating part of the lip and restricting the vibration of the lips.

There should be a pressure point on the lower teeth as well, because the lower jaw is the strongest bone in the body and can absorb great amounts of pressure, and the part of the lip that is the source of vibration is the center of the upper lip, and this part needs to be protected by overbalancing the pressure toward the bottom lip, away from this critical area.

Teeth structure is one-third of the proficiency in the higher register. The other two-thirds consist of the proper use of the embouchure muscles and the proper use of air. With the possession of the pressure point on the top and bottom teeth, the proper use of the muscles and air, and proper practice over an extended period of time, it is possible for a trumpet player to increase his range to include double high C and above.

SYMPHONIC SOUND AND ATTACK

Symphonic sound has a darkness and more centered quality of sound than the brighter, lighter sound of the virtuoso style and is accomplished by making the oral cavity a little larger, deepening the "ah" sound by dropping the back of the tongue, and by moving more lip into the mouthpiece, thereby increasing the vibrating surface of the lips. The result is the characteristic darker, more centered sound.

The notes are also stretched in order to play with proper symphonic style. The symphonic attack is accomplished by building up the air pressure and delaying the release of the tip of the tongue, which causes a firmer, sharper initial attack.

TRANSPOSITION AND CLEF STUDIES

Transposition and clef studies, particularly important for orchestral trumpet players, are taught by the use of the clef or interval systems, depending on the preference of the student. This skill involves the study of the tenor clef by trombonists, and includes the understanding of the techniques involved in transposition and practicing appropriate exercises that help develop these skills for all players.

SIGHT READING

The important faculty involved in sight reading is the ear. The purpose of the eyes in sight reading is to identify the sounds that the ear hears. The key to developing this skill is to look at a passage and immediately transfer what is seen into what would be heard. Think of sight reading as: "When it looks like this, it sounds like this." The main way to develop this skill is to be mentally aware of the fact that it is the ears that are reading, and not the eyes. The concentration on and development of this mental skill incorporated with the proper use of appropriate reading exercises gives the student the potential of becoming a fast, accurate sight reader.

The 14 skills worked! Students progressed faster, Jerry spent less time correcting problems during band rehearsals, the kids glowed with their newfound confidence and the greatest critics, parents, were pleased with the results.

If Jerry taught students already involved with their school music programs, he supported their band directors and helped students with skills during private lessons.

When on tour and a parent asked him what to look for in a teacher, he said, "If you can find someone who can tell you how to do it and also show you, that's a super teacher. If you must choose between the two, go for the information. One who says, 'Here's what you do to make it sound like this.'

"But when it comes to practicing," Jerry would go on, "remember the practicing is to gain control over the muscles and to develop your skills to a subconscious reflex. You can't set a time limit on that kind of practicing."

To a student seeking a professional career he would say, "If you're skillful enough and go where the action is, you can make it. But you have to develop the skills. If the trumpet is between you and the music, you'll never make it.

"If you're contacted to do back-up work and this commercial is costing hundreds of dollars a minute, you'd better have the skills to go in there, read the music and play. If you can't do that, the director will say, 'Hey, I don't have time to let you learn how to play' and you're out the door."

In his constant quest for ways to help his students, and to improve his own performance, Jerry developed an interest in teeth. When he was still in Pennsylvania, he'd been unable to play in the extreme high range, and he wanted to correct that. So he observed and studied those who had command of the skills he wanted to develop.

Hitting high notes, Jerry reflected, depended on fast vibration of the lips. If the teeth were too flat, the pressure of the mouthpiece against the teeth could cut off circulation, and that would make vibration and high tones impossible. He'd heard of musicians who'd had teeth moved to help range. Maybe that was what he needed.

Jerry started visiting orthodontists. Most of them didn't understand embouchures and the components of range – teeth, air pressure and lips. And they certainly couldn't see any reason to spoil nice, flat teeth for some musician who was essentially instructing them in what should be *their* expertise. They declined and bid him "Good day!"

Then Jerry met Dr. Lester Gordon, an orthodontist in McKeesport, Pennsylvania, who had achieved some success with moving the teeth of the Shiners, two brothers who taught at Duquesne University. Dr. Gordon declined to do Jerry's teeth because they'd been weakened by diabetes. But Jerry considered the meeting with Dr. Gordon helpful because he learned that Gordon was forming teeth into a wedge with the use of full braces and a retainer. He started referring his students to Gordon.

When Jerry moved to Winona Lake, he looked for a local dentist to help his Grace College students, worked with Eugene Dellinger, a Fort Wayne orthodontist, for a while, and then settled down with Dr. Thomas Van Osdol, a Warsaw dentist. Van Osdol, who helped students with braces, retainers and crowns, also hated to see good teeth ground down for the expensive capping process, but he soon came to understand the importance of the process to future careers and earning capabilities.

But then Dr. Gordon entered the picture again, with a development that made both Van Osdol and Jerry happier. Dr. Gordon was using a hard shell overlay to correct overbites. Jerry, who asked Gordon to send one to Warsaw so he could study it, was intrigued by the device. It was just a piece of clear plastic for the lower teeth, but if it were turned upside down and a wedge molded into it, maybe they could use it on the top teeth. Jerry drew diagrams explaining how the wedge should be shaped and took it to Van Osdol.

Van Osdol, using normal methods for making plastic dentures, took an impression, made a mold and poured plastic into it. After a dental lab provided the cuts, sanding and shining of the overlay, he fitted and adjusted it in the mouth of the musician. He was pleased. It didn't spoil teeth, it was inexpensive, removable and it provided the bumper effect that Jerry sought.

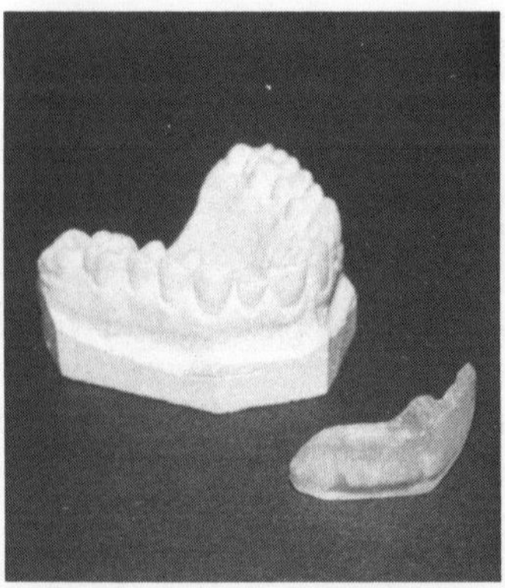

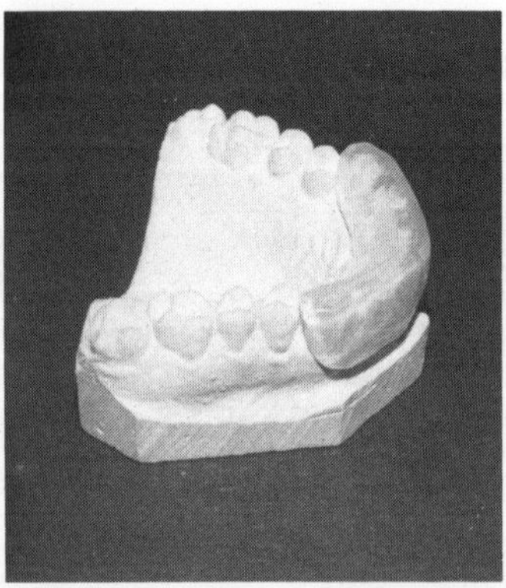

Overlay and plaster model

Jerry was pleased too. High C still evolved after much practice, but with the overlay the lips were protected and could function to full capacity. "Just like a bumper," Jerry quipped to a student. "It protects your grill."

Soon students and professionals, hearing by word of mouth and by reading about it in *Tic* and *The Instrumentalist* magazines, were contacting Jerry for consultation and an overlay. Tom Richeson, of the Diana Ross Show, sought overall competence. He spoke with a teacher who referred him to Doc Severinson, who in turn referred him to Jerry. Jerry Sadbury of New Mexico wrote, seeking information and expressing his pleasure about "the first printed article dealing with musicians' dental problems that I have found."

Musicians were excited about the development. Some described the overlay as "the most dramatic thing to happen to brass in modern times." Jerry simply called it "helpful for the person who doesn't have the natural endowment."

Ken Brader, lead trumpet and assistant music director of the Glenn Miller Orchestra, didn't have the natural endowment. He heard about Jerry through Phil Norris, a former Franks protege, and from Parke Frankenfield who had read about Jerry through one of the magazine articles. Brader visited with Jerry, but found that he could not spare time to adjust his embouchure to the overlay because he was on the road 50 weeks of the year. He did, however, receive help from Jerry, who showed him how to shift the pressure point to his left front tooth to get the most out of the teeth he had.

From overlays, the next step in wedging musician's teeth was bonding, a procedure whereby teeth were ground down, cleaned, and covered with repeated plastic layers. It took about 30 minutes, was not removable and achieved the same effect as braces and overlays: better tone, increased range and greater endurance.

Endurance was what Jerry needed in the late '70s. He was directing and traveling with the Dimensions in Brass, teaching 90 students a week, traveling for Conn, and helping students and musicians with their teeth. But not helping himself. He was out early, up late; meals were haphazard, often snacks and the forbidden sweets that he loved. His family was concerned.

"Don't push yourself so hard," said his brother Mickey.

Dottie cautioned about his eating. His mother urged him to get a check-up.

His father pleaded with him. "Don't do what I did. Look what I did to my heart. I had to have open-heart surgery. Don't you do this kind of stuff."

But Jerry was doing what he enjoyed, what was worthwhile. He didn't argue, he just kept going. The first sign of trouble came in the summer of 1977. Jerry and Dottie had built a new house, a tri-level in a woods near the college. Jerry, Dottie and Rich Dick, a student, were painting the interior of the house.

"Boy, Jerry, you may be a musician, but you sure aren't any good as a painter."

"What do ya' mean? I'm a highly experienced painter. You learn all kinds of trades when you have to live on a teacher's salary." Jerry's laugh was a deep, infectious chuckle.

"Well, if you played the horn the way you're painting that baseboard, you'd be on welfare."

Jerry looked closely at the baseboard, prepared to fire another wisecrack at Rich. But on close examination, he found that Rich was right. There were heavy blotches on some spots, and no paint at all on others. Maybe he needed to have his glasses checked.

A few days later, Jerry, his children, and a friend, Wilmer Witt, were on their way to the stock car races in South Bend. Jerry was driving. It was a dark night, made worse by a pouring rain, but U.S. 30, a four-lane highway, cutting east and west across northern Indiana, was well marked.

Suddenly, car lights, the center line and pelting shards of rain were lost in a black blur. Jerry gripped the steering wheel, searching for the flared area of light ahead of the car. Where was the center line, the edge of the road? He knew they were still moving forward, but without the speedometer, a vision of road and car, he couldn't gauge their speed.

He had a terrible anxiety for the safety of the people in the car. He should pull off the road. But where was the side of the road?

"Dad–" a breathless warning came from the back seat. Dad, what are you doing? it said; Dad, watch out! it said.

"I can't see!" Jerry cried.

Wilmer Witt didn't ask questions or wait for an explanation. He grabbed the steering wheel. "OK, Jerry, I have it. You can brake gradually and I'll guide us to the berm."

Tense quiet pervaded the car, as everyone concentrated on the move from road to berm, from speed to standstill. Even after Wilmer and Jerry had changed places and they were moving down the highway again, the car was quiet, as each occupant pondered what had happened.

As his sight returned, Jerry thought that maybe what he'd experienced was like a white-out or disorientation brought about by rainy night blending into gray road and dark landscape . . . or maybe he needed a change of glasses. The next day he called Dr. Richard Carman of Warsaw, and made an appointment.

At the end of his examination, Dr. Carman turned on the lights, made a few notations on a chart, and rolled his stool over to the large hydraulic chair where Jerry was sitting.

"Jerry, what I'm seeing is that you have a few ruptures in your right eye that are interfering with your vision."

Ruptures, Jerry thought. Diabetes did things like that. "Probably caused by the diabetes, huh, Doc?"

"Yes, that's a possibility. I'm going to make an appointment for you with an ophthalmologist. He can evaluate your situation better than I can. But I'm sure it's nothing to worry about."

The Goshen ophthalmologist, Dr. Troyer, sent Jerry to Dr. Markstone in Indianapolis. The consensus was that "it was nothing to worry about; it would clear up."

But during a trip home from Omaha in the fall of 1977, Jerry was detained in O'Hare Airport in Chicago. Planes were stacked up over the airfield, waiting for a hole in the weather so they could descend. Jerry had to stay alert, keep his eyes on the screens announcing flights in order to know when his plane landed and was ready to take on passengers. But the screen wouldn't stay in focus. The tiny lines of letters blended together, making it difficult for him to discern flights and times.

By the time his plane finally landed in South Bend, his sight had deteriorated so badly that he needed help in deplaning. But again, the next day, his sight had cleared.

The next bout with blindness occurred at Christmas time, when he and his family were returning to Uniontown to spend the holidays with their families. His eyes failed and remained obscured until three days after Christmas, when he awoke with full vision.

In Warsaw, after the holidays, Dr. Moser examined him. There was no trace of burst blood vessels – only pink, healthy flesh in his eyes. Dr. Moser said, "I can't see any sign of a rupture."

But Jerry was beginning to think heavy thoughts. His eyes had been gone three days this time, three days of feeling his way, of listening instead of looking, of relying on others. What if he went blind for good? How could he make a living for his family?

There was only one way he wanted to make a living: teaching and playing music. Maybe he should memorize his methods books, "just in case."

For the next three months, during lessons, during free time, whenever he could, Jerry concentrated on capturing the printed page in his mind. He also took care of another, important kind of business. He wrote a love letter to Dottie. He had never written one before, so he decided it was time to put in writing what he felt.

On several sheets of lined notepaper, he gently, tenderly told her how much he appreciated her joyful attitude, her help through the ordeal with his eyes . . . "What you don't know is how much of a source of strength you have been to me. Many times, when I have been on the verge of getting down, or feeling sorry for myself a pleasant smile, or a hug or squeeze from you was all it took to make my spirits soar again . . . I truly believe that you are what the Bible describes as a virtuous woman, and I shall cherish you for the rest of my life."

Jerry folded it twice, put it in an envelope and left it on Dottie's pillow. It was the last thing he wrote before that eventful Easter Day of 1978.

Chapter 6

That Devil Diabetes

8:00 a.m. Late November 1980. Century Center, South Bend.

Coats flying open, two representatives of Bach Instrument Company hurried across the parking lot to the car where Jerry was sitting. They'd been told that Jerry couldn't do his solo for the meeting of The Association of Christian Schools International and that he could not move from the car because of a nosebleed. They were not prepared for the scene that met them in that car.

Jerry was in the front seat, head resting against the cushions. His suit, white shirt, the cloth he held to his face and the seat were splotched with blood. On the floor, his badly swollen feet rested loosely in his untied shoes.

"Jerry, what can we do?" they asked.

"Nothing, I'll be OK. But maybe I'd better not plan on doing the concert."

"When did it start? Here? In the car?"

Ellen Berghorn, Jerry's secretary, turned troubled eyes to them. "It started this morning at the motel. We used towels, *everything* to stop it. We thought we had it under control, but it started again when we got here."

"Jerry, you'd better see a doctor."

"No. It'll be OK. I'll just lie down for awhile."

"Well, we'll cancel the workshop too."

"No, that's not until 3:30. I'll be able to make that."

"Are you sure?"

"Yeah, I'll see you later."

When the flow of blood finally ceased at 2:30 in the afternoon, Jerry rose, shaky and weak, and returned to the Century Center. There he found that he had to rest after every few steps in his climb to the second story. He had to conduct the demonstration and clinic while sitting down, in order to perform at all.

In the car on the way back to Marion, dizzy and almost at the end of his strength, Jerry thought about the situation. The last two years had been marked by change and health problems. First, in the spring of 1979, there had been the terrible pain in his right eye. It had felt like a huge cinder resting on burned flesh. Dr. Steve Grossnickle, Warsaw ophthalmologist, had diagnosed glaucoma and suggested a less than serious solution.

"Well, what works with things like this is marijuana. I can let you smoke 'pot.' "

"Yeah, that would be great," Jerry had joked. "I can get an incense burner and sit in my office over at Grace College and smoke pot."

Grossnickle had prescribed Timoptic and Diamox, a diuretic used to reduce intraocular pressure, right before Jerry and the Dimensions in Brass left for a European tour. The diuretic had affected Jerry very badly. He'd become so lethargic that he couldn't stand. And then there had been the tomato juice incident; the kids had teased him about it for months. While riding on the bus in Germany, he'd been drinking tomato juice, had felt a sneeze coming on, but had been too "out of it" to pull the container away from his face. The eruption sprayed juice all over his face and the surrounding area. Jerry smiled to himself in spite of his fatigue, as he remembered that day.

He'd stopped taking the medicine, but then the pain had come back. Great pulsing waves of pain.

"An ulcer in the eye," Grossnickle had said. "You can't take this pain. On a scale of one to ten, your pain is a nine. I think it might be a good idea to take your eye out and put in a glass eye."

"No," said Jerry. "Medical science may have given up, but I haven't given up on God, and God can't heal a glass eye."

"Well then, let's try freezing the eye and after that, using Timoptic again."

The freezing and Timoptic had worked; he'd had no

more trouble with the eye. But then the fatigue had started. He'd attributed it to their spring 1980 move from Grace College, to building a new home in Gas City, Indiana, and to getting established in a new teaching position at Marion College at Marion, Indiana.

Marion College, a small, coeducational, community college founded in 1920 by The Wesleyan Church, reposes among the busy, shaded streets of the city. Its goal is to develop the minds, souls and bodies of young people.

Marion College officials knew about Jerry Franks. Dr. Robert R. Luckey, president of the college, had heard him play at a benefit for ministers in Winona Lake. So, when Marion College administrators faced a vacancy in the music faculty and heard that Jerry was thinking of making a job change, they hurried to invite him to join the faculty.

Jerry's arrival at Marion College had introduced a kind of hubbub that Marion had not experienced before. Many of Jerry's Grace College students transferred to Marion; professional musicians buzzed in from time to time for lessons; and music educators came seeking advice on the purchase of instruments and choice of music schools. Marion College accepted and enjoyed the change, negotiating to preserve a well-rounded musical diet and also to allow Jerry to perform the music he enjoyed.

It had been a good move, Jerry thought, but he could have enjoyed it more if he hadn't been so tired all the time. Little by little, he realized now, his energy had declined. By summer of this year, weakness and fatigue sat on him like an overweight albatross, pressing down, making every action an effort.

Dr. Moser suspected anemia, and had tried several types of iron supplements to combat the problem. He'd also made urgent pleas for testing. Jerry had been "too busy," and anyway, anemia ran in his family. A shot of B12 was probably all he needed.

Then new afflictions descended: the swelling of his feet and legs to grotesque proportions, and a cold and congestion that caused great difficulty in breathing. He'd told Dottie not to worry. The swelling in his legs was probably because he was sitting so much, he didn't get enough exercise. And the cold? That would go away.

He had to admit, however, that he'd never had a cold that caused so much trouble. He couldn't sleep because he couldn't breathe lying down. And on the way home from his dad's funeral in Uniontown just a week before, he couldn't get his breath as they drove home.

Eyes, fatigue, congestion and swelling, and now a seven-hour nosebleed! All things considered, Jerry decided, it was time to call Art Moser.

When Moser saw Jerry the next day, he wanted to check him into the hospital. "We'll give you some transfusions to get your blood count up and run some tests."

"I can't, I have too much to do," said Jerry.

"Well, how about this Friday then?" Moser countered. "We could check you in for the weekend, do the tests . . ."

"And I'd be back in school on Monday?"

"Yes. We could run the tests we need over the weekend."

"OK, but I have to be back on Monday for classes."

Stubborn Franks. That's what Jerry's mother called the Franks clan. They wouldn't "doctor" and they wouldn't take care of themselves; if they had something they needed to do, they'd forget how they felt and get the job done.

That was Jerry's attitude too, but he checked into Kosciusko County Hospital on Friday, November 28, for the testing. The seven-hour nosebleed had done it.

That Friday evening was "old home week" at the Kosciusko County Hospital. Area friends, learning that he was in Warsaw, came by to see him. As usual, there were a lot of jokes and laughter.

"So, they're working you so hard down at Marion that you need a vacation already, huh, Jerry?"

"Well, at least, I *worked* for three months. When I was at Grace, you were on vacation all the time!"

When Jerry called his mother, he said "Hi, Mom, I'm in the hospital." He laughed. "Don't worry, they're going to give me some blood, probably some B12 and some diuretics to get the swelling down. It'll be OK."

Two days later Jerry had gone from jaunty and laughing to silent and immobile as he sat in a wheelchair and listened to Dr. Moser.

Moser spoke quietly. "Jerry, it's a kidney problem. It didn't show up in the other tests we did, so I didn't suspect it. But this last test showed that it is the kidneys."

Jerry and Dottie listened attentively. There was something in Moser's face, Dottie decided. Was it sadness? Yes, and grief, as if he were telling someone a friend had died. But his words were casual: "kidney problems."

Moser went on, "What we're going to do is transfer you to Lutheran Hospital in Fort Wayne. They can care for you better there. And they'll put you on a dialysis machine and dialyze you a couple times . . ."

It was decided that Moser would call Lutheran and make the arrangements for admittance, and Dottie would call Rob to drive them to Fort Wayne. As they were finalizing the arrangements, Moser, a friend of the Frankses, gave Dottie a gentle hug and again Dottie noted a restrained sadness in his face. But she was too occupied with getting Jerry to Fort Wayne to think about it very long.

She didn't think about dialysis much either. It was what Max Brenneman had had after kidney failure. That was all the word meant, a term that applied to someone else's experience. Besides, she was worried about Jerry; he wasn't talking, he wasn't moving. In spite of her lack of knowledge about dialysis, she felt a fearful urgency to get him to Lutheran as soon as possible.

Jerry, for his part, was not aware of too much that was going on. All he was aware of was vomiting suddenly and violently without feeling sick – one of the symptoms of kidney failure.

Kidney failure can be caused by polycystic kidney disease, glomerulonephritis (inflammation of the filtering units of the kidney), diabetes, or high blood pressure, which cause the buildup of metabolic end products in the blood and result in uremia.

Jerry was suffering with uremia and had been for some time, the earliest symptoms being anemia and fatigue. Then came severe uremia with its nosebleeds, and after that end-stage renal disease with its swollen ankles and shortness of breath.

The people at Lutheran knew what they were dealing with. When Jerry was established in his room, he was put on oxygen and given diuretics.

Jerry wondered briefly why they had put him on oxygen, and then slipped into oblivion again. Meanwhile, Dr. John Dyer, nephrologist, called Dottie into the hall. He was honest with her.

"Jerry has end-stage renal failure . . ."

Dottie looked into Dr. Dyer's blue eyes. They showed concern, compassion. Dottie felt secure to have Jerry in this gentle man's care.

"That's uremia that has gone as far as it can go," Dyer continued. "His kidneys aren't functioning, so there's been a buildup of the fluids that should be excreted through his urine. That's why his feet are so swollen and his breathing is difficult."

"He's been bothered with that for weeks!" said Dottie.

"I'm sure he has. The truth is, Mrs. Franks, Jerry is critically ill. He's in danger because the fluid he's retained is causing stress on his heart. Congestive heart failure is the problem right now, but we'll do everything we can."

"Can I stay with him?"

"Certainly. We'll have a couch brought in."

As Dottie watched orderlies bring in a black couch and place it ceremoniously against the wall, she thought, black couch. Same color as my pants and sweater. Same color as the night and my feelings. Then she waited, listening to the pulsing, gurgling machines establish a rhythm that beat like the tick of a clock. Pulse . . . pulse . . . pulse . . . pulse. She found herself breathing in time with it. Pulse . . . pulse . . . pulse . . . pulse. Helping Jerry live. Willing Jerry to live.

Then she remembered all the people who wanted Jerry to live. His mother, oh, his poor mother! She'd just lost a husband. How could Dottie tell her a son was near death too?

Dottie talked to her children briefly, explaining what Dr. Dyer had told her. She called Mickey, Jerry's brother, and asked him to call his mother, and then she returned to Jerry's room. Dr. Dyer was already there, established in a chair beside Jerry's bed.

While the hours slipped away in half-lighted night, to the accompaniment of pulsing machines and swishing nurses, Jerry awoke periodically and wondered why the doctor was staying so long. They had said kidney failure, but all he knew was a fatigue so encompassing that the only reality was the bed, its supporting softness and his total reliance on it.

"How are you doing, Jerry?" Dr. Dyer was beside him.

"OK."

"Can you breathe?"

"Yeah."

Then Dottie was beside him, her hand on his hand. "I'm here, Honey."

But the weakness was unbelievable, the bed not soft enough or deep enough to relieve his fatigue. He couldn't answer before he slipped into darkness again.

Dottie stood beside the bed awhile and then went back to her cot. ". . . critically ill, in danger . . ." kept repeating itself in Dottie's brain. Why hadn't they seen the symptoms?

Jerry had always been a night owl, coming home from a lesson at 9:30 p.m., staying up with the late movie and then rising early, chipper and happy. But for the last year and a half, he'd come home and fallen asleep. In fact, when he wasn't at school or teaching lessons, he was asleep. Why hadn't she seen the drastic change?

And his legs and feet, so swollen he couldn't put his shoes on at a family wedding earlier in the month. How could they have thought it was only because he held a job where he got no exercise? He'd been doing the same thing for 14 years and his feet hadn't swollen!

And the "chest cold" . . . he couldn't get his breath, even when the wind was in his face in the car.

As Dottie pondered and questioned in the darkened hospital room, her mother-in-law, Kitty Franks, and her brother-in-law, Mickey, were traveling the nighttime roads of Pennsylvania and Ohio on their way to Indiana.

Mickey had called Kitty to say that Jerry was very ill and they needed to leave right away. Rev. Clyde Landrum at Warsaw had called too and told her that Jerry had been transferred to Fort Wayne. Kitty was shaken. She'd just buried her husband, and now Jerry was sick. But Kitty decided she would not fall apart. She couldn't be of help to anyone that way. She'd gathered her clothes in a bag and was waiting when Mickey arrived.

The next day the sun came out both inside and outside the hospital. Oxygen, diuretics and transfusions had turned the tide. Jerry was breathing more easily and he was able to respond to his weary, relieved family.

Then Jerry was taken to dialysis to remove the poisonous toxins in his blood, and dialysis became more than a word, a procedure associated with their friend Max Brenneman.

The doctors and nurses prepared them quickly: dialysis was necessary for life and would continue as long as Jerry lived or until a transplant donor could be found. And Dottie – if she chose – could be the one to administer the procedure.

The first day, Dottie observed the procedure, learned about shunts, fistulas and the awesome care that must be taken to ensure sanitary conditions. She was to learn much more later.

The two methods of getting blood from the body to the hemodialysis machine and back to the body are the shunt and the internal fistula. The shunt consists of two small tubes that are inserted in the forearm. One is inserted in an artery and another in a vein nearby. The internal fistula consists of an artery connected to a vein so that blood is carried directly from the artery to the vein; during dialysis, two hollow needles can be inserted in the veins and, after attachment to tubes, carry the blood to the dialysis machine.

The fistula is preferred over the shunt because the shunt requires great care and cleanliness to prevent infection or injury; but the fistula takes several weeks to be ready for the entry of needles, so a shunt is used until the fistula is ready.

Thus the first order of business two days after Jerry was stabilized was the insertion of a shunt.

Dr. Michael Schatzlein was a surgeon *and* a trumpet player. He had met Jerry when Jerry and the Dimensions in Brass recorded albums at Schatzlein's TRC Studios in Indianapolis. He knew the special needs of a trumpet player.

"Hi, Jerry. It's Mike Schatzlein," he said as he entered Jerry's room.

"Hi, Doc!" said Jerry. "How are you?"

"Just great! I hear you need a little hardware in your arm."

"Yeah, I guess so."

"Well, when I heard that you were here, I said 'I know that guy; I'd like to do the shunt for him.' "

"Hey, that's great!"

Shatzlein moved closer and touched Jerry's arm. "Listen, I've been thinking about this. I got out my old horn, played it and tried to figure out which arm would be the best to put the shunt in. What I've decided is that the left arm would be best. It would hamper your playing the least, and you would be less likely to work the bandage loose and get infection in it."

"Sounds good to me."

"Then when we put in the fistula, we'll put it in the right arm, OK?"

"OK."

When Dr. Luckey, president of Marion College, visited, one of the first things Jerry said was, "Hey, you know what?"

"What?" said Luckey.

"My doctor is a trumpet player and he figured out how to put the needles in so it doesn't affect my playing!"

"That's wonderful, Jerry!" said Luckey. "But don't worry about getting back to work. You just get well. We'll get along until then."

Jerry was at Lutheran Hospital three and a half weeks. While doctors experimented and adjusted the dialysate mixture to find the best one for him, Dottie began her three-month course in preparation for doing home dialysis. The nurses, Lisa, Barb and Jane were special. Their zany antics – one time a soft-shoe and song in goofy hats – lightened the atmosphere; their warmth and kindness made dialysis less stressful.

There was stress enough for Dottie. For one thing, she thoroughly disliked anything mechanical; for another, she'd heard stories of the difficulties of dialysis and the stress on the dialysis partner. Would she run from the building as Elaine Brenneman had when she first witnessed a "run"?

Dottie didn't run when she was first ushered into the dialysis unit, but she did experience a moment of panic. The throbbing machine, cold, metallic, with all its pulsing tubes and fluttering gauges seemed menacing to her. Seemed to be daring her to learn its secrets.

I can't do-o this! Dottie said to herself. But almost immediately there came an inner voice that said, "I can do all things through Christ which strengtheneth me," and calm and confidence settled over her once again.

When she took her first look at the "SET-UP PROCEDURE FOR DRAKE WILLOCK #4215 USING HOLLOW FIBER DIALYZER, she couldn't believe the number and complexity of the dialysis steps.

1. Drop concentrate line into bottom of proper

concentrate jug. (Make sure end is hitting bottom of jug.)

2. Make sure rinse flag is up over conductivity meter.

3. Turn Drake on. Press rinse button on inside of machine, left side. Press reset button.

4. Make sure:
   a. Pressure gauge on right side of R.O. is 20-40.
   b. Pressure gauge on left side of R.O. is 150-210.
   c. Rocker arm is moving.
   d. Flowmeter is at 500cc/minute.
   e. Negative pressure is between 25-50.

5. While conductivity is coming up:
   a. Thread arterial line through the blood pump, making sure the sidearm is on the right.
   b. Make sure the line is snugly against the wall of the blood pump.
   c. Clamp airway on arterial bubble trap and attach 10cc syringe.
   d. Turn arterial bubble trap upside down and place in holder.
   e. Knot off heparin line. If using heparin pump clamp off heparin line.

   (Conductivity should now be up in the safe range of 90-120mEq/L. An alarm will sound and your conductivity and rinse light will go out. When this happens, push rinse flag down – alarm will automatically stop.)

6. String venous line:
   a. Place venous filter right side up in air level detector.
   b. Place empty jug on top of machine.
   c. Open blue cap on end of venous patient line and place in top of empty jug.
   d. Depress arm on line clamp, thread line through line clamp.

e. Connect Swinnex filter to positive pressure gauge.
f. Connect monitor line snugly to Swinnex filter.
g. Clamp monitor line close to venous filter tightly using shodded fistula clamp.
h. Place Harvard clamp on venous patient line below line clamp.
i. Clamp airway and attach 10cc syringe to the end of airway.

She stopped reading and leafed through the pages. There were two more pages like that, not to mention the numerous pages of the BEFORE GOING ON CHECKLIST, the huge print CHECKLIST FOR PUTTING ON THE SHUNT, the AFTER GOING ON checklist and the huge print AT TIME TO COME OFF instructions.

Unbelievable! How would she ever master all that? It seemed impossible. But – she said to herself – Lisa said she would have three months to learn it. She'd just take one step at a time.

The steps were myriad. She had to learn the process from beginning to end: getting supplies from a closet, hooking up all tubes, filters and machinery, testing the machine, and running saline through it to clean the lines. Then, after Jerry was attached, adding drugs to the dialysate – the liquid mixture that washed the blood and carried insulin, and the blood-thinner heparin and other substances. She had to take "coags" – a testing of the coagulation properties of the blood and chart weight, blood pressure, temperature and machine pressure. And she had to know the procedural problems of dialysis: black blood, blood leaks, hypotension (abnormally low blood pressure), infection and incorrect dialysate concentration.

She learned to wrap the shunt and Jerry's wrist after dialysis. With great care and precision, she would slip one edge of a 4″ x 8″ gauze pad under the shunt openings, fold the pad over the top and then with strip gauze, wrap shunt and arm firmly so no foreign matter could get near the shunt openings.

She came through her training with flying colors, dispelling any insecurities she may have had about her ability to handle "mechanical things."

There were other things that Dottie and Jerry had to handle, however – some dark statistics about diabetes and dialysis. Because of the fragile state of a diabetic's health, a diabetic on dialysis had a life span of about three years. Many dialysis patients, who felt sicker on dialysis than without it, were unable to work because of fatigue and debilitation; many marriages collapsed under the stress of a situation with little hope. And some patients, feeling so ill, with no hope and no real life except moving from bed to chair to bed and back again, simply chose to die.

Social workers and counselors informed Jerry and Dottie of the emotions they might have. Like those in the grieving process, dialysis patients often experienced denial, anger and depression, especially if the crisis was totally unexpected. Patients often cried, Why me? refused to take responsibility for their own care and railed at doctors and nurses, or, absolutely loathing attachment to and reliance on the machine, walked out of the hospital, never to be seen again.

Some other facts were that dialysis removed waste up to only 10-15% of normal kidney action and could not correct anemia, blood pressure and blood sugar problems.

Jerry and Dottie listened, but they refused to dwell on the negatives. For Jerry it was simple. He called upon what he had believed since childhood: "God is real, Jesus Christ is alive and cares for His own. We're placed here to serve Him and He's going to help us." It was what had gotten him through blindness; it would get him through dialysis until a transplant was available.

Chapter 7

Dottie

8:00 a.m. A morning in 1981.

"Boy, isn't this great!" Jerry spoke from the recliner in the Frankses' family room. "Not to have to get up at 4:00 a.m. to go to Fort Wayne to dialyze?"

"Um-hmm, sure is, Honey." Dottie was adjusting a tube at the end of the dialyzer.

She'd just moved the rectangular, metal dialyzing machine to Jerry's chair and started the saline solution through the lines. It was still new to her. She'd had three months of training under Barb, Jane and Lisa, but now she was on her own and she needed to concentrate.

Pulling on tight surgical gloves and shaking peroxide on a cotton ball, she reviewed the preliminary steps with the aid of the instruction book on the coffee table to the right of the machine: "Remove the plugs from the shunt; wipe the opening of the artery tube away from the vein tube; with a new ball, wipe the vein tube away from the artery tube. Repeat the process with Benadine and Benadine ointment. Don't want any bacteria in the tubes when you start."

She attached the tubes of the machine to the tubes of the shunt in Jerry's arm and straightened. It *was* good to be at home. To take only five hours Monday, Wednesday and Friday instead of five hours plus two hours travel time to Fort Wayne. She'd organized her Marion College schedule so that she could get most of her classes on Tuesdays and Thursdays. But some had to be scheduled for Mondays, Wednesdays and Fridays, so being close to Marion was a big help. It was another help to have Jerry's shunt still working. Most clotted off within three months, but Jerry's was still good, so she didn't have to punch large needles into his arm every time.

As she watched the blood course through the tubes from Jerry's arm to the dialyzer she wondered what kind of a run Jerry would have. Would the machine maintain the right amount of fluid to prevent leg cramps and itching? Could she keep the heparin level stable?

She had to take great care. Every run was a life and death situation – death if Jerry didn't have dialysis, death if he did and bacteria or cleaning solution were left in the lines or machine. She had to watch gauges and filter levels to be sure that there was the proper mix of oxygen, saline and blood. She had to keep Jerry awake so he could let her know how he was feeling.

Blood, one of God's miracles, was the life-giver, life-carrier. It kept the body fed, cleaned and stabilized, but when it was removed, its flow or components disrupted, all areas of the body were affected. There could be leg cramps, vomiting, unbelievable itching, even unconsciousness and coma, because of sudden, violent drops in blood pressure. Dottie always entered the dialysis process with conscientiousness and meticulousness.

She watched the flow, the clear saline solution entering Jerry's arm and the red blood leaving the other tube in Jerry's arm. She noted the color of the blood. If it turned black, there was formaldehyde in the lines and she'd have to act quickly to shut off the blood pump and clamp the blood lines.

Her eyes followed the thin line of red as it went through its checkpoints, climbed to the dialyzer on the right and came out the other side. The Venus filter, which was the last checkpoint before the flow completed its cycle, had to be watched constantly at the beginning, to gauge whether the blood level in the filter was too high or too low. If the blood level was too low, air entered the line; if too high it could pop the seal on the filter.

As Dottie watched, the blood level inched steadily upward. Seems pretty high, she thought. Oh no! It's getting too high! But it was too late. The top flew off the filter and the buzzers and alarms shredded the air.

"Oh no!" Dottie cried aloud.

"What's wrong?" asked Jerry.

Blood was spewing out the top of the filter, falling like rain on Jerry's prone figure, plinking thin rivulets on the metal dialyzer cabinet and spraying a mist of droplets on the pages of Dottie's instruction book, obliterating letters and making an alien language of the words printed there.

"What's that?" asked Jerry.

"Don't panic, that's your blood." She didn't feel as assured as her voice sounded, but instinct took over and she clamped the flow from the filter.

"What's wrong?" Jerry asked again.

Dottie was too busy to answer. Popped filter or not, they still had to dialyze Jerry and that meant starting over. But his blood was in process, how did she get him off to start over without losing his blood? She'd have to call Fort Wayne.

"Jerry," she said, "I've got an emergency. I can't talk right now. I'm going to call Lutheran."

Dottie peeled off the surgical gloves, dropped them in the garbage can that stood near the dialyzer and strode to the phone, where she recoiled when she touched the receiver. Blood! Clear over here?

After dialing the hotline number for dialysis patients, she listened anxiously then said, "This is Dottie Franks at Gas City. We have an emergency . . ." She described the problem to Lisa.

"OK, turn off the . . ."

"I've already turned off the blood pump and clamped the blood line," said Dottie. "But I don't know how to get him off the machine!"

"OK, Dottie. Is anyone else there?"

"Yes, Jeff's here."

"Give the phone to Jeff and I'll talk you off."

"I'm worried, Lisa! The blood is black and I still have to dialyze him."

"It's OK, Dottie. That's because of the lack of oxygen. Don't worry, just throw away the blood that's in the machine."

"OK, here's Jeff."

Jeff calmly relayed Lisa's instructions to Dottie, who step by step turned dials and closed lines until she'd managed to bypass the machine and get Jerry unhooked. Then she had to start all over again, which meant removing and replacing all the tubing, putting on gloves, preparing the shunt tubes, taking off gloves, putting on new gloves, connecting the tubes of the machine to the tubes of the shunt. Gloves, swabs and gauzes, tubes and seals accumulated in the garbage can near Jerry's chair, as she went through the process again.

Later, she wrung out the last bloody cleaning cloth and leaned against the sink. A factory defect, a broken seal, was the problem. How could she have known what to do for that emergency? The people at Lutheran didn't expect it to happen. Still, it had worked out all right. She hadn't panicked; Jeff had been there and Jerry had waited quietly in his sticky, blood-spattered clothes, not screaming at her or chewing her out for her mistakes.

She had full understanding of why marriages crumbled under the stress of dialysis. It was a frightening, debilitating, often painful procedure. Jerry, immobilized four hours, exhausted, in pain when too-dry tissues caused leg cramping, could very easily become impatient and fearful and yell at her. And she, under the stress of maintaining his life by drawing blood for "coags," administering drugs and keeping watch over gauges and tubes, might have grown bitter and angry.

She admitted to some "wishing" occasionally: that Jerry could see so he could watch the gauges, that he could take his coags and clean his own machine like other patients, but she didn't get bitter and angry.

She didn't and he didn't. He lay quietly, patiently, as the machine pulled his life's blood out of him, cleansed it and pumped it back again. In an emergency, he listened, waited and did not add to her concern. He accepted, just as he had accepted the fact of permanent blindness that day in April 1978.

He and Rob had returned from their visit with an opthalmologist in Michigan, the third doctor consulted after Jerry had gone blind. That event, indelibly painful, was, by comparison with present happenings, a quiet place in her memory. It was the only time she'd had the luxury of thinking how she was feeling as the crisis was in progress.

She'd been in the roomy kitchen of the house in Winona Lake, the last child of her day care group had left, and she'd just dropped spaghetti into a pot of boiling water, when Jerry and Rob entered the room. Jerry found his way to one of the benches at the trestle table and sat down. Rob paced quietly behind him. Father and son both had peaceful countenances. Jeff and Marcy joined them.

"Well," Jerry said. "The bottom line is I'm going to have to learn to live my life as a blind man. The doctor says I won't see again."

Dottie stirred and stirred, as realization and sorrow washed over her. Never see again? No blue skies, flowers or . . . She lifted her head as if to find an answer and her eyes locked with Jeff's. Jeff's eyes, so much like hers, were full of pain and disbelief. How could this happen? they seemed to say.

Yes, how could it happen? It *can't* be happening, she thought. Things were out of control, crazy. Jerry blind!

She stirred and stirred, watching the pasta strands wrap around her spoon. I should turn down the heat before I go to the bedroom, she thought.

In the bedroom, as in most instances of grief, she'd wept for more than one loss. She'd cried for Jerry, for Jeff, for all of them.

And now, in the little house in Gas City, Dottie remembered the long ago and present sorrows and wept again, for the lovely, roomy house, the friends she'd left behind, for life as it had been.

She sighed, straightened and gave herself a mental upbraiding. You're thinking negative thoughts, she said to herself. Remember, you're supposed to talk nice to yourself.

Though Dottie believed that "the steps of a good man are ordered by the Lord" and that their move from Winona Lake had been ordered by God, she still found the change a difficult one. In Winona Lake, the Frankses' house had been a "central station" of doors slamming, phones jangling and neighbors popping in. Her children and their friends, the children of the day care classes and the students from the college traveled in and out, bringing all the happy bustle of numerous people and their activities.

In Gas City, a small town south of Marion, the whole scene changed. Rob had stayed in Winona Lake, in their unsold former home. Jeff at Marion College and Marcy, a junior at Mississinewa High School, were in school all day. All was quiet. She had no small children to help break the ice with mothers of other small children. She had no day care to bring adults in, and her old friends were over an hour away. So Dottie had decided to go back to school and work on her degree in elementary education.

Then, two months after the start of school, Jerry's kidneys had failed and Dottie had been thrust not only into a new house, but a new lifestyle and a new role. She had to be nurse, coach and the boss of the family. It was unfamiliar territory for her. She wasn't sure she was making the right choices. But "give in" was never a part of Dottie's vocabulary, so she went on, and she learned the meaning of chronic illness.

Chronic was long-time, continuous. And continuous described kidney failure. There was no reactivating a destroyed kidney. It might be bypassed, its work taken over by dialysis; but the consequences of a dead kidney were always there: no cleansing of the blood; the imperfect results and side effects of dialysis; the need for a donor kidney that would match. Chronic illness stretched before her like a long, black tunnel with no light at the end.

It was a difficult time for all of them. Rob had held down a job and also driven hundreds of miles to take them to Fort Wayne, Indianapolis and back to Gas City again. Jeff, with his terrible disillusionment about God and why He let this happen to his dad, was a walking wound. Marcy hated her small room, and she and Jeff were both appalled at the changes that kidney failure had brought, in their lifestyle and in their father. He was actually stingy, talking about "cutting back" all the time, and uncharacteristically, blowing up when they asked him for a little extra money.

Dottie understood that Jerry wasn't always able to think as clearly as before. Dottie understood the pain that Jeff was carrying and Marcy's distress. She understood all of them and carried the burden of their pain, along with her own pain and distress at not being able to make everything right again.

She prayed for them all and kept going. If there was any help for them, it was the Lord, who promised to be with them always, "even unto the ends of the earth." That was certainly a promise for chronic illness.

As Dottie emptied the ten-gallon garbage can of swabs, cotton and tubing, she remembered what had led to her "mental fitness formula." It had been a day like this several months before, when she started to leaf through a stack of bills.

Keltsch Pharmacy – dialysis supplies . $1,992.25

Rental of dialysis machine, one month . $600.00

She had stopped. It was staggering! There were bills for doctors, for travel, supplies. Marion College had a very good Blue Cross plan, but that alone couldn't cover the $30,000 to $35,000 yearly cost of dialysis. They'd applied for Medicare; but though Jerry was one of the first diabetics eligible under a new Medicare plan, they didn't know if he would be accepted.

There had been some well-timed helps to their financial situation. The house in Winona Lake had sold at exactly the right time – when Jerry was in the hospital with kidney failure. And they'd been able to return to the builder their new split-level colonial in Gas City and move into a small house. But the economic reality was that they still had no way of knowing whether they would make it or not, or what they would have in the future.

Jerry's health was stabilized, but little by little, unconsciously, his body was eliminating activities that weren't necessary. He slept after school, after meals and between lessons. With the three-day-a-week dialysis and his increasing inertia, his teaching schedule was interrupted, his private lessons decreased. Would they lose that income altogether?

The spring concert tour was coming up. Could he do it? And what about his clinician work with Conn? That required a lot of travel and playing – and energy! She'd gone back to school, but graduation was years away. What was ahead for them?

Her mind had spun from thought to thought, until she'd felt there was no hope, no sense in getting up the next day to face it all over again. No end. There was no end to the dark tunnel.

And then the alarms had gone off in her mind. She could imagine them to be like the alarms on the dialysis machine, flashing lights and a shrill beep, beep, beep, beep. Warning, warning! Malfunction!

Yes, she'd thought. That kind of thinking was a malfunction. It was the kind of thinking that made for mental illness and desperate deeds. She had to do something to help herself, to somehow get a hold on things. She'd prayed for guidance and then gone to the bookstore to arm herself for the battle.

What she'd found engendered a lot of introspection and self-evaluation: "The most common cause of depression was a sense of being trapped, unable to remedy an intolerable situation."*

Well, that certainly described a family under dialysis – restricted, hemmed in by the constraints of time, money and energy. So she wasn't alone; many people were depressed by such a situation.

"The primary cause of depression is self-pity."

Was that her problem? Maybe. It was difficult not to play "poor me" from time to time. She had to worry and figure to pay the bills; she had to make decisions about the children; she even had to do the things that other dialysis patients did for themselves. And the "coags" – she hated to do the "coags." And she disliked taking apart the machine piece by piece and cleaning it. Yes, she did feel sorry for herself occasionally. But what could she do about it?

The books said that she could choose happiness, choose to rest in God's power.** Of course! She knew that! But initiating the thinking was very difficult when there were so many problems.

Well, she wanted to have *something* under control, and choosing how she would think and whom she would rely on was certainly a form of control. Maybe then, resting on God's power, she could manage the strength to go forward a little each day and get to the end of that dark tunnel.

The books gave the steps she needed to follow and she adopted several that she found helpful.

1. Change the way you talk to yourself.
2. Understand your feelings, but focus on behavior.
3. Focus on a specific plan of action.

With her decision to choose what she would think, Dottie had taken the first step. When the "poor me" thoughts take over, she reminded herself, you're thinking negative thoughts. The Lord wants you to think on true,

---

**How to Win Over Depression,* Tim Le Haye

***Happiness is a Choice,* Frank B. Minieth and Paul D. Meier

honest, just, pure, lovely things. He doesn't just say these are "nice" things, He says *think* on these things.

So the good news was that Jerry was alive, she was healthy, there was hope of a transplant, they had a home. When she started thinking of the pluses, she found that they went on and on.

Understanding her feelings and the causes of them helped her to see that fatigue made her vulnerable to negative thoughts. Realizing this, she could remind herself that she would feel and think better after a good meal, a night of rest or some little bit of recreation.

The specific plan of action Dottie adopted was to make lists of long- and short-term goals and to cross off the items as they were accomplished. Checking off each item helped her see where she'd been and what she'd done. It gave her the sense of control she needed and provided victories over two old problems: lateness and procrastination. With the aid of her lists, even the hated charting and bookwork of dialysis was dispatched and crossed off quickly.

In her kitchen now, on this morning in 1981, Dottie reached for her list for the day. Above the first item she drew a long arrow to the right side of the page and turned the sheet over. Then she made a new list.

1. Dialysis, watch the blood level rise in the filter.
2. Panic (briefly).
3. Call Lutheran.
4. Reroute Jerry off the machine.
5. Replace all tubing and seals and start over.
6. Dialyze.
7. Replace all tubing and seals.
8. Remove garbage can very full of surgical gloves, swabs, tubing and seals.
9. Discover the distance that blood under pressure can travel by cleaning it off Jerry's chair, the table, machine, walls and behind pictures.
10. Rinse bloody cloths.
11. Lean against sink.
12. Be sad.
13. Think on good things (a sense of humor doesn't hurt either!).

The items of good report were that she, the "Little Woman" type of wife who hadn't driven a car until after Jerry's kidney failure, was learning a new self-confidence.

Three days each week she held her husband's life in her hands, and each time she preserved it.

The good things were that Jerry was OK, patient and trusting; that Jeff, who was normally in class at that time of day, had been there to help; and that Lisa, one of the wonderful people at Lutheran, had been quickly available. The final item of good report was that the Lord was watching over all of them!

With quick, sure strokes of her pencil, Dottie put a check mark beside each item, turned the sheet over so that her original list was visible, and went to the family room to check on Jerry.

Chapter 8

"Since I Look Like Dad, Will I Be Fat Someday Too?"

Spring 1982. On tour in Florida.

". . . anyway, after I went blind, we went on to Iowa, where we did 25 more concerts. If you ever go blind, Iowa is a good place to go, 'cause there's absolutely nothing there *to see.*

"When we came back, I went to the doctor and he said, 'You're blind!' and charged me forty bucks!

"Then he said, 'You'll have to do something else for a living; you can't possibly direct and play because you'll be too dizzy and you could fall off the stage and hurt yourself.' I said, 'What am I going to do about the 25 concerts I've already played?' You know, people are so nice. Here I am lying on my back playing away and nobody even said anything.

"Then, in 1980, I lost my kidneys. I was just walking across the parking lot and they jumped out and took off. Now, if I could have *seen* I coulda' grabbed 'em . . ."

Jerry was sharing his story, his tongue-in-check version of blindness, kidney failure and dialysis, with the audience.

In the band behind Jerry, Jeff and Marcy Franks watched the people in the audience as they smiled, chuckled and then laughed aloud at Jerry's jokes.

Jeff and Marcy did not smile. Marcy's eyes were dark with fear. Jeff, a wry twist to his mouth, was thinking, We have the unfortunate privilege of knowing what's going on.

Jerry was dying, that was what was going on. And

they had front-row seats on his fight for life. At home, at school, on tour, they watched Jerry teach and sleep, perform and sleep, eat and sleep. He was awake only long enough to do the most necessary activities.

But Jerry was determined to go on. "I'll strap the machine on my back if I have to," he'd said.

He did not strap the dialysis machine to his back, but he did send blood samples and instructions to dialysis centers in the towns where he and the Dimensions would be appearing. The results were not always satisfactory. The run that day had been a bad one, leaving Jerry totally drained, so that it had been necessary for Jeff and Marcy to support his bent, staggering body as they entered the church that evening. They'd exchanged worried glances that said, He'll never make it through the concert tonight!

But Jerry had pulled himself upright at the last minute and proceeded, playing his horn, telling his jokes and giving his testimony. Jeff and Marcy knew that as soon as the concert was over Jerry would wilt again. It was the pattern of his life now. The doctor's predictions were coming true right before their eyes: "A diabetic on dialysis has a life span of about three years." Jerry was well into his second year and getting steadily weaker.

Fear was a black weight on their lives, crushing the hope out of them. The repeated crises fell on them one after another, each blow tempering a steely surface over the churning fear and despair inside them.

Jeff couldn't understand why these things should happen to his dad. His dad was a good, honest person. He knew lots of people who deserved it more. It wasn't fair!

Marcy awoke every day expecting to learn that her father was dead. Every phone call struck a death knell in her heart. While trying to imagine how she could ever handle Jerry's death, she wished fervently that her father had never become ill, that things could be as they had been before the kidney failure.

Rob, Jeff and Marcy were born in 1960, 1962 and 1963 respectively. They all remember that their mother was always there, their father seldom there. He went to work before they left for school; he came home after they'd gone to bed. But when he was at home, he was available to them.

To Rob, Jerry was somehow bigger-than-life. Wherever he was, that was the place to be, for his kids and his students. Jeff remembers that Jerry wrestled, played ball and went to the races with them. Marcy, proud to be Jerry's "little Mugsy," loved to lie on the floor beside him, watching TV or rough-housing with him and her brothers.

Jerry's position as Director of Instrumental Music and Artist-in-Residence, his prominence in the music world, provided a special dimension to their lives. There was continual activity and an occasional game partner because of the college students who gravitated to the Franks house. There were the recognition and privileges of being "Jerry Franks's kids." And all three loved it. "After all," as Jeff put it, "if they know him, they're gonna feel better about me. Why should I mind that?"

Jerry's blindness had created no major problems in their lives. He had to be chauffeured wherever he went; but Rob, 18, and the students at the college didn't mind an opportunity to get behind the wheel. Other than the driving, things went on the same. Because Jerry was accepting of the blindness, he was as he'd always been: joking, good-natured and caring. So the children, after the initial shock, took cues from him and accepted it too.

But the kidney failure and dialysis destroyed the balance of their lives, sending them into a wobbly, whirling orbit where everything was upended or thrown apart. Financial security was destroyed, life was not guaranteed, parent was child and child was guardian.

Rob, a realist, who displays an aspect of easy imperturbability, was out of high school, staying in the Frankses' Winona Lake home and working at Nellans Motors in Warsaw when Jerry entered the hospital in November of 1980. The plan was that when Jerry had had all the tests prescribed by Dr. Moser and KCH personnel and had been released, Rob would drive his mother and father to Marion.

But when Rob went to the hospital on Sunday evening, he'd noticed Jerry's deteriorated appearance. To Rob, Jerry looked as if he'd aged 10 years. He wondered how the doctor could release his father when he looked so bad. Rob soon learned, however, that the destination was not Marion, but Fort Wayne.

In the car on the way to Lutheran Hospital, Rob, disquieted by his father's gray, sunken face and incoherent answers, suggested that they stop and get an ambulance. But after discussion he and Dottie decided that it would be better and quicker to continue to Fort Wayne – at top speed.

Jeff and Marcy in Marion were expecting their parents' arrival when Dottie called.

"We're going to take Daddy to Fort Wayne, to Lutheran Hospital."

"What? I thought he was being discharged," Marcy answered.

"Doctor Moser says that Daddy has some kidney problems."

"Will he be all right?"

"I hope so. He's not looking very good, but Moser says he just needs to be dialyzed a couple of times – you know, like Max Brenneman. Listen, I have to hurry, Honey. Why don't you and Jeff drive to Fort Wayne?"

Questions and confusion dominated Jeff's and Marcy's thinking as they drove to Fort Wayne. Dad had gone in for a routine check-up; he was supposed to be back at school on Monday morning. What had happened in two days' time?

When they arrived at Lutheran Hospital, they were greeted with even worse news.

"Dad has congestive heart failure . . ."

They were stunned. "How . . ."

"His kidneys have failed because of the diabetes, and the fluid has built up, affecting his heart."

"But he was fine when he went into the hospital!" Marcy wailed.

Dottie shook her head slowly. "We just didn't understand the symptoms. You know, nosebleeds, swollen legs and congestion?"

Marcy and Jeff stared at their mother, unbelieving.

"Doctor Dyer says that tonight will tell; if he's all right in the morning, he'll be OK."

That was all the information that Jeff, Marcy and Rob received. Their mother went to Jerry's bedside and they settled in in the hospital lounge. To Jeff, slouched on the sofa, looking at the TV, but not seeing it, it was a nervous time. The message they'd received from their mother and the doctor was "hang out and fake it." In other words, wait till morning and see what happens. That was easier to say than do.

For Rob, it was stepping off the hours, pacing out his tension, thinking it ironic that other kids were always fighting with their dads, wanting to get away from them. And he who didn't understand such feelings and had never felt a need to escape, was in danger of losing his dad permanently.

Marcy was struggling with numbing disbelief. How could her dad die because of a cold, nosebleed and swollen feet? What had really happened? What if he died? She didn't want him to die.

There had been a time when she'd wished she didn't *look* like him when she'd been about five. Because everyone told her she looked like her father, she'd assumed that her stomach would swell and she'd be fat like her dad. She had drawn pictures of herself with a huge stomach and written her name beside them. Finally, she'd asked her mother, "Since I look like Dad, will I be fat someday too?"

Marcy had been infinitely relieved to learn that she wouldn't grow up to be fat. Now, she decided, she wouldn't mind looking like her dad if he could just be OK.

In the morning there was good news and bad news. Jerry was stabilized, he would be going on dialysis, but he would never be completely "OK" again.

Doctors at Lutheran knew that patients whose kidneys failed unexpectedly had greater difficulty adjusting to the demands and discomforts of failure and dialysis, so they informed them of what they would face, if possible, *before* they faced it. They also informed the family in the hope that knowledge would help minimize their shock and confusion.

Red-haired Dr. Dyer sat down with Jerry's family, leaned toward them and, fixing kind blue eyes on them, carefully explained the problems.

"Jerry will be on dialysis until we can find a kidney transplant, but dialysis isn't perfect. It can do only 10-15 percent of what the natural kidney can do. Because of that, no one can live on dialysis indefinitely, and a *diabetic* on dialysis has a life span of about three years.

"Jerry is an excellent candidate for a transplant," Dyer added quickly, "so we'll put his name on the list." Dyer studied the faces before him, took a breath and continued.

"I would be remiss, however, if I didn't tell you that even that is no guarantee. Jerry's health might not be good enough to undergo surgery, and if he can, the transplant might not stay. It's a tough prognosis, and not what I *expect* to happen. I just have to let you know all the possibilities."

Lutheran personnel, aware of the possibilities for emotional trauma, informed the Franks family about the availability of psychiatric help with some of the problems they might encounter. Family roles would change. Instead of Jerry, the parent, being strong and supportive, Dottie and the children would have to support Jerry. Such changes would be frightening, and would create conflict and anger over the loss of personal time and the alteration of their lives.

A lowered hematocrit could make Jerry tired and impatient and contribute to a personality change that would confuse and anger his family. And Dottie, needing to devote large portions of her time to Jerry's care, would have less time to meet the needs of her children.

On top of all that, there would be the overpowering fear of death, and the terrible, all-consuming wish that Jerry could be well and things could be normal again.

The upheaval began almost immediately. Rob, who would be removed from most of the day-to-day anxieties because he lived in Warsaw, was pressed into service as driver. When Jerry was released from the hospital, he and Dottie had to return for dialysis and home training. Dottie didn't drive, so Rob arose at 4:00 a.m. – every day at first, then three days a week – drove to Marion, picked up his folks and took them to Fort Wayne. Then he returned to Warsaw and went to work. After dialysis, Jeff picked up Dottie and Jerry and drove them back to Marion.

Some weeks, Rob was required to go to Fort Wayne on Monday, Indianapolis on Wednesday and Fort Wayne on Friday. So some days Rob would go to Marion, to Indianapolis, back to Warsaw and to Indianapolis and Marion again. For Rob it was "a hard way to make a living."

It was also a lean time financially – for Rob, who spent a good part of his salary on gas, and for his parents who were drawing on savings and making hard decisions about their financial future.

The new two-story colonial-style house in Gas City would have to go! They'd only been in it a few months, but they couldn't pay dialysis charges and make large house payments too. So, abruptly, they asked the builder to take the colonial house back; they found a small house in Gas City and moved.

Abrupt. Jarring. From a lovely, roomy new home, the children were transplanted to a very small, unpretty house close to a busy street.

For Marcy, this was crisis number five. First, there'd been the lengthy, name-calling sessions by a misguided high school administrator at Winona Lake; number two was the death of her beloved Grandfather Franks one week before number three, Jerry's kidney failure. Number four was the frightening prognosis about Jerry's health and number five was financial reversal and another move to a new house and a new school.

She felt as if she were being pounded. Boom! "You're no good." Boom! "Grandpa's dead." Boom! "Daddy can only live three years on dialysis." Boom . . . boom . . . boom!

It was useless to care about anything, better not to be happy, because something bad would happen if you were. Constantly tensed, waiting for the next blow, she envisioned herself to be like a surface that was continually pounded – resistant and hardened.

But she was not resistant; the pain and worry were still there. When she tried to study, she saw reruns of the scenes at home, and homework seemed trivial compared to the life-and-death activities she witnessed every day. When her friends became worried and her mother asked her if she wanted to see a psychologist, she said no. She knew they couldn't afford it anyway.

Included in her emotional turmoil was guilt. She resented the responsibility put upon her, but felt guilty when she was resentful and angry. This is your father you're talking about here, she would say to herself, cut him some slack!

To Jeff, everybody was "nerved out." The financial strain, coupled with the effects of dialysis, made Jerry uncharacteristically irrational. A request for gas money elicited a volatile response and provoked an argument, and then Jeff would argue with his mother and Marcy about why he shouldn't argue with his dad.

Adding to the strain were the clamorous alarms on the dialysis machine, Jerry's appearance and inertia, and his insistence that he would keep going no matter what.

Jeff had a philosophy of helpful forgetfulness; when an incident was over he thought, good, that's over, now I can forget it. And he *would* forget it. But he found that there weren't any stopping places with kidney failure and dialysis. There was no vacation from the tension, and worse, the worry about death.

Rob, in Warsaw, expected to hear bad news all the time. He admired Jerry and Dottie's positive attitude and their ability to think better of people than they were, but he knew Jerry was being unrealistic. When his dad surprised everyone and kept going in spite of all odds and the fatigue he suffered, Rob knew how he'd done it. "The Lord had *every*thing to do with it!"

Then, early summer of 1982, two months after the trip to Florida and two weeks before Marcy's high school graduation, a new bad thing happened. Jerry developed the restless leg syndrome. A condition caused by impaired conduction of impulses down the nerves, and more severe in diabetics than in other dialysis patients, it produced twitches at 8- to 12-second intervals and made it impossible for Jerry to sleep. After a depression induced by Seconal and other central nervous system depressants prescribed to relieve the syndrome, Jerry had to endure drug withdrawal.

Jerry felt like he was going to explode. His mind and body could not rest. He and Dottie would sit on the front porch, where they would try to enjoy the fresh air and soothing motion of the swing, but Jerry could not sit still. He would shift positions repeatedly, stand up, pace the few steps across the porch and then tell Dottie he wanted to walk around the block. When they got halfway down the block, he would turn around and go back. After swinging a couple of times he would need to walk again. The procedure was repeated again and again.

For Dottie, it appeared that Jerry's mind was racing. He was like a record or movie played at fast speed, his speech fast and garbled, his actions rapid and uncontrolled. Dottie adapted herself to his needs, walking when he needed to walk, talking or listening when he needed to talk. The days of August 1982 were not measured in 24-hour periods, but in the severity or lessening of Jerry's reactions. When withdrawal was complete, and it was time for school to start, Jerry was weaker and more emotionally spent than he had ever been.

The rest of the family was spent too. That fall the Chinese water torture of crises falling on them threatened to bring them to the breaking point.

One more thing . . . one more thing . . . one more thing. Jeff was tired. It was to be expected. When events piled on one after another, it catches up with you. But it shouldn't be expected that his dad should have to suffer all those things. Why did God let it happen? Why wouldn't He heal his dad?

Marcy, always waiting for the next blow, anguished every time the phone rang in her dorm at Marion College. One ring was an in-house call; two rings meant an outside call. Whenever there were two rings her heart stopped. She was terrified that it might be bad news about her father.

These feelings were aggravated by Jerry's behavior. Students reported that he fell asleep during lessons. In rehearsals, he would give instructions and the downbeat and then say "just play", totally uncharacteristic of the man who usually conducted – with the flick of a finger or lift of an eyebrow – every dynamic of a musical number. And when Jerry was in his office with nothing demanding his attention, he slipped into a half-conscious condition, eyes closed, barely breathing. Marcy, who helped as Jerry's secretary, watched and worried. Was he breathing? Would this be the day? But then a student would enter or a class time approach and Jerry would draw from some obscure reserve of strength to do what was needed.

And that too was a problem for Marcy. Because Jerry revived when needed, few people knew how dangerously close to the edge he was and could not understand or sympathize with Marcy's pessimism and fear.

By mid-November of 1982, Jerry was so weak that he couldn't lift his arms to direct. He was suffering with constant backache and he was considering making an unheard-of concession to his feeble condition: he and his students were discussing how he might conduct and perform while seated in a chair.

Jerry, Dottie, Rob, Jeff and Marcy, pounded and weakened, worried and angered, but still recognizing the sources of strength to be family and God, pulled together. They kept their fears and worries to themselves in order not to make Dottie's load any heavier. They helped each other: Rob came running when Dottie called; Jeff came running when Marcy needed help; Marcy sympathized in Jeff's dark moments.

They were frightened. They knew that Jerry couldn't go on much longer, but they never forgot the greatest strength of all: God. Dottie prayed fervently for a kidney donor; Jerry asked for prayers from his students; Rob recognized that the reason that Jerry was able to navigate at all was that God was helping him; Marcy knew that the only people she could count on were God, herself and her family; and Jeff, though he'd questioned God, knew – as he'd written for a 1980 *Guidepost* Youth Writing Contest – that Jerry's illness was a witness to others.

Jeff had seen their faces, the woman thinking of suicide; the man going to prison; the man on dialysis in Fort Wayne. They'd looked at Jerry as if he'd put gold in their hands. Maybe that was why his dad was able to continue; God wanted to show how He could bring triumph out of a person's life, no matter how human or sick he was. God could reach through that illness and say, "See, here I am. I can help you too."

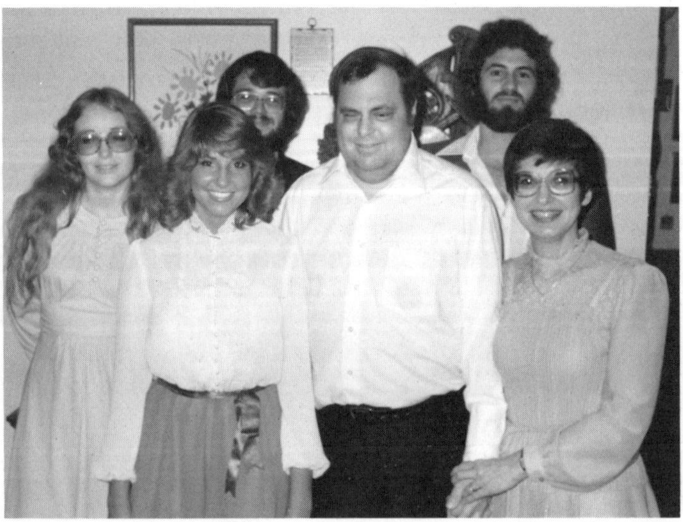

Family picture at Marcy's high school graduation. L to R: Jerlene (Rob's wife), Marcy, Rob, Jerry, Jeff, and Dottie (1982)

Chapter 9

"A 24-Year-Old Kidney"

5:40 p.m. Mid-November 1982.

Ethel Shaffer, Dottie's mother, was alone in the Franks home when the jangling of the phone startled her. There was high hope that one day soon a phone call would bring news of a kidney donor. She hurried to the phone.

"Hello?"

"May I speak to Jerry or Dottie Franks, please?" said a woman's voice.

"I'm sorry, they're not here right now. Is there a message?"

"No, I have to speak to Mr. or Mrs. Franks."

"Is there a phone number where they can reach you?" asked Mrs. Shaffer.

"Yes. And would you please tell them this is an emergency."

Mrs. Shaffer copied the number, trying to contain her excitement. It was the renal division of the Indiana University Medical Center in Indianapolis. Maybe it was the transplant!

Five minutes later, Dottie arrived.

"Oh, Dottie," Mrs. Shaffer waved a paper in the air. "Here's the number. It's an emergency!"

"It's Jerry's kidney!" Dottie jumped up and down and hugged her mother. "I was sure they'd find one."

Events moved very quickly after that. Dottie called

the number and was told to be at the hospital in Indianapolis by 7:00 p.m.

"Now, I want you to realize," said the nurse in Renal Transplant, "if the tests show that there's no match, you may have to take him back home. But come prepared, because if it's a match, he'll be hospitalized."

Dottie called Marion College, where Jerry and Jeff were rehearsing with the Dimensions, and told Jeff to bring his dad home right away. Jerry had to be in Indianapolis by 7:00 so the kidney could be transplanted within 24 hours after removal from the donor.

Marcy, at the women's dorm on campus, did not have to endure the double ring of the phone that brought her news about Jerry. She was at dinner in Baldwin Center when she was paged for a phone call. A page was as frightening as a double ring, she found, because a page meant there was an emergency.

"Hello?" she asked. What is it this time? her hello said. Is it good or bad?

"Marcy? This is Jeff. Dad got a kidney. I'll pick you up in five minutes."

Marcy returned to the table. Breathless, stunned, she tried to tell her friends about the kidney, but she couldn't speak past the lump of emotion in her throat.

After a flurry of happy hugging, packing and phone calls, the Frankses were finally on their way to Indianapolis. But as the car sped along the dark highway, Jerry, in the back seat, was having second thoughts.

Did he really want to do this? Dialysis wasn't perfect, but he was getting along OK. Well, not really OK. But he would have to spend a minimum of 30 days in the hospital. What would his family do while he was recuperating? His salary paid for the bills, utilities and house payments, but the day-to-day expenses – gas, food and extras – came from the private lessons he taught. If he was laid up for 30 days and more, how would his family manage?

Adding to Jerry's concern were the depressing facts about transplants. If there was even a hint of infection in his body, they wouldn't do the surgery at all; he would have to go home and wait for another donor. As a diabetic his chances for success were lessened. He might die on the operating table. He could spend hours on the table and have the kidney reject right away, or, after going through the surgery and recovery, he might not live a year.

Dialysis had left him drained, and it couldn't correct his anemia or blood pressure problems. But it was familiar, and like all human beings, Jerry feared the unknown more than the known devils.

"Dottie?" said Jerry tentatively.

"Yes, Honey?" said Dottie from the front seat.

"I don't know if this is such a good idea."

Dottie was quiet a moment, then she spoke carefully. "Oh, I think it is, Jerry. You've been very fatigued the last few months, right?"

"Yeah, I guess so."

"Haven't felt like doing much at all, right?"

"Well–"

"Well, we have to take a chance. The Lord hasn't brought you this far to let you down now. We just have to trust. OK, Honey?"

"Yeah, I guess."

Doubt surfaced again when Jerry lay on a hospital table for four hours, waiting for the results of tests. But Dottie stayed beside him, encouraging and reminding him of the positive aspects of the procedure. Then Dr. Ronald Filo and Dr. Guier, a resident, came in.

Renal transplant specialists walk a fine line. When they enter a patient's room after testing, they're speaking to a person who's tense from the rushed trip to the hospital, and relieved because a transplant is finally available, a person who's hopeful for a return to an every-day, before-dialysis kind of life, and scared about surgery. Such heightened emotions often make it difficult for a patient to assimilate the information the doctors must impart.

But impart it they must, and, while maintaining a positive attitude, they must help the patient and family understand the risks and alternatives.

"We have a half match," said Filo. "A half match means that it is more normal than abnormal. Only a perfect match does better."

Dottie squeezed Jerry's hand, her eyes sparkling with sudden tears.

"And that's real good for you," continued Dr. Guier, "since you're diabetic. Diabetics do better with a transplant than with dialysis."

"We must inform you about some things, however."

"Yeah, I know," said Jerry. "Dr. Dyer told us that there were some bad points and I'd hear more about it here."

"That's right, Jerry. You could die on the operating table, but it's unlikely. You may not live a year. The kidney may reject so that we'd have to take it out and you'd have to go back on dialysis – but weaker than ever because you've just had surgery. You're a diabetic; that increases the risk. So! That's the story. Now you have to make a decision."

Jerry and Dottie had acquired quite a knowledge about kidneys, dialysis and transplants by this time. The kidneys, which carry the largest blood flow of any organ their size, are, like the blood they filter, another miracle of life. About four inches long and two inches wide, they are composed of hundreds of thousands of tiny nephrons which accept and send on the substances needed by the body, rejecting the waste substances, which then go to the ureters and bladder.

The reserve power of kidneys is tremendous! When one normal kidney is removed, the remaining normal kidney enlarges and increases in function by approximately 50 percent and functions at approximately 75 percent of both kidneys.

Kidneys, which clean the blood, and maintain the body's chemical balance, have no peer. Dialysis, with its pumps and filters, functions at 10-15 percent of the efficiency of a kidney and cannot maintain the chemical balance or correct for anemia, high blood pressure and blood sugar. Dialysis is risky for a diabetic, the side effects more severe. But the transplant, though it functions better than dialysis, is never fully accepted by the body. With the help of steroids, the body accepts a "truce" with the strange intruder, but never stops trying to reject it.

Still, if they were to transplant, it was best to transplant as soon as possible. That was what Dr. Dyer had told them. Certainly this was "as soon as possible." Jerry and Dottie decided to go ahead with the surgery. The Lord had helped all along the way; they had to trust that He would continue to help.

At 2:00 a.m. Jerry went into surgery. His faith was rewarded with a kidney that worked, even before he left the operating room!

As often happens, however, the kidney rejected about

five days after surgery, giving Jerry and Dottie personal knowledge of the capricious blood components, creatinine and BUN, the poisonous end products that need to be expelled from the body.

A two-week regimen of ATG serum was prescribed to combat the rejection. Administered in a five-hour IV drip, it caused terrible weakness, heavy sweating and body-quaking chills.

In the middle of all this strife, there entered a bit of sunshine. Thanksgiving Day, Jerry, on the bed, and Dottie at the window were contemplating Thanksgiving without family. Dottie, wanting to allow Jeff and Marcy a respite from hospital and anxiety, had encouraged them to accept invitations from friends.

Then, quietly, there appeared at the door, Lois and Jack Hardin, Dottie's sister and brother-in-law. Lois studied her sister a moment. Dottie, her face in profile, was pensive, an aura of softness about her that touched Lois deeply. How she must feel, thought Lois. Thankful for Jerry's transplant, yet yearning for past years and family all around her. And she's so small, her shoulders too narrow to carry so many burdens. But she'd continued on, not complaining, just doing what had to be done. Lois was filled with pride in this "little sister" of hers.

Then Dottie turned and saw them. Smiling, she hurried toward them. "You came!" she said. "And on Thanksgiving!" She hugged them, eyes shining with tears.

There was no table heaped high with food that day, only hospital trays of turkey and dressing. And instead of a house full of family, there were four in an austere, white-washed room; but the meaning and heart of Thanksgiving were maintained completely: family gathering in thankfulness, supporting one another in love.

A change in the administration of the rejection-suppressive drugs brought another ray of sunshine to Jerry and Dottie. The second ATG IV was administered more slowly, and Jerry's blood chemistries progressed toward normalcy.

But then Jerry encountered another, more benign problem of recuperation: boredom. Dottie and his mother were with him, they talked, they read, they talked some more; but Jerry, who shakes a foot when he can't be busy and active, did a lot of foot shaking.

In December, when it was time to go home, Jerry

was dismayed to hear that he had to rest for three months more!

"But I'm scheduled to teach J-Term. Can I do that?"

Doctors Filo, Leapman and E. J. Smith had heard this kind of thing before. Patients were often over-optimistic about recovery, but full recuperation had to be assured. "When does it start?"

"In January."

"That's an awful short three months."

"If I get better real fast, can I do it?" asked Jerry.

"Well, you're going to have to get awfully good awfully fast. We'll see."

When J-Term time came, Jerry asked his doctors again. "Can I teach that course?"

"You're immuno-suppressed, you know."

"Yeah, I know. My white blood cells are suppressed by the medications I'm taking, so they can't help me fight off colds and other stuff."

"So you'd have to wear your mask and not be around people with illness. Could you teach the course at home?"

"I could probably work that out."

"OK, since you're doing so well, and *if* you wear your mask, and your students wear masks if they have even the hint of a sniffle, then we'll let you teach the course at home."

When J-Term started, Jerry, in a white hospital mask, stood in a circle of students in the family room of the Franks home.

"Hey, Look! It's the Lone Ranger!" said one student.

Another hummed the "William Tell Overture."

"You know, it's the strangest thing," said Jerry. "When I walk into the bank with my mask on, everyone gives me money."

What Jerry could not see that J-Term was that the room was often dotted with "mysterious masked men" who practiced imaginary quick draws and deadeye shots at each other.

When he and Dottie made their first visit to "Clinic," the periodic check of blood and urine chemistries at I.U. Med Center, Dottie was glad that Jerry couldn't see.

As Dottie guided Jerry through the main entrance and up a flight of stairs at Long's Hospital, she was thinking how well things had gone. After the rejection, Jerry had improved rapidly and had been able to leave the hospital on schedule, 32 days after surgery. Not like the poor man who had "rejected" just before dismissal and had to start all over again! Jerry looked good too. He'd been out of the hospital four days, he was down to 158 pounds, and he was joking again.

"Wait a minute, Jerry, these doors open toward us." She stopped, pulled on one of the double doors and led Jerry inside. "OK, Honey. It's a long hall, no obstacles."

As they progressed, Dottie noticed the people moving from room to room. One woman, one hip lower than the other, walked with an irregular gait; her cheeks looked like she was storing nuts for the winter. There was a man with huge stomach and a swollen face covered with acne; a woman with bloated stomach, swollen cheeks and neck, and painfully thin arms and legs.

Dottie paused. Where were they? Did they have the wrong floor? The wrong building?

"What's the matter?" asked Jerry.

Dottie watched a large man approaching. Thick hair covered his hands and arms, and protruded from his ears and down the side of his face. What had happened to these people?

"Dottie?" The question was in Jerry's voice.

"It's OK, Honey. I'm just trying to figure out where we're supposed to go."

Thirty-eight people were at the clinic that day. A large number for one clinic, a prodigious showcase of the side effects of the steroids that prevented transplant rejection.

Renal transplant personnel had told Dottie and Jerry about the side effects of steroids and other immuno-suppressive drugs: cataracts, ulcers, gastrointestinal hemorrhage, lowered immunity to infection, weight gain, appetite increase, bone changes and hair growth. To Dottie, that first clinic day, "side effects" was translated "deformity"!

But Jerry was Jerry again. Instead of the lethargy and withdrawal of pre-transplant days, Jerry was teaching, directing and joking with the old verve.

"Hey, I'm feeling great! I've been thinking, I'm gonna call Bo Derek, maybe Lonnie Anderson . . .

"Yeah, why not? I've got a new 24-year-old kidney, so I'm subtracting 20 years from my age for my new kidney. Hey! I'm not gonna stay married to a 44-year-old woman when I'm only 24."

Jerry soon resumed a full teaching load at Marion College and recommenced lessons with the students of all levels who traveled from around the state and from other states. In addition, professionals like David Evans, a studio musician from Los Angeles, popped in for lessons, consultation and bonding.

Although Jerry still had to travel to Indianapolis or Fort Wayne once a week for checks on blood chemistries, it was a far easier schedule to manage, because he didn't have to juggle lessons and classes around three mornings of dialysis.

Administrators of Marion College were always supportive of Jerry, visiting, encouraging and reassuring him. It had long been their goal to achieve a level of excellence commensurate with non-Christian schools, so they were pleased to have Jerry, his expertise, and teaching ability.

They found his philosophical and emotional attitude remarkable. He lived his faith, carried his load, ill or not, and he did outstanding public relations work for the school. In the community of Marion, Jerry and the Dimensions in Brass performed for groups like the Mississinewa Art Council, the Marion Philharmonic and the Rotary Club – a normally stoic group that gave Jerry an unprecedented standing ovation.

When the college needed recruiting help, Jerry was involved. When donations or interest waned in supporting churches, the college "pulled out all the stops" two or three times a year and sent Jerry. It was a compatible partnership.

Jerry had a peaceful co-existence with his transplant too. He'd developed a few of the side effects of the medications he was taking: hair growth, enlarged stomach and thickening neck, but he compensated with larger clothes and open-necked shirts. Under Dottie's watchful eye, he took his medications and insulin and ate what a diabetic should. His visits to Fort Wayne and Indianapolis became less and less frequent.

But Dr. Dyer was concerned. He was not only concerned, he was on the horns of a dilemma. Always, at the earliest opportunity, he talked to renal patients about keeping a positive attitude, not giving up. And here was Jerry with such a positive attitude that he was maintaining a schedule that was endangering his life – in Dyer's estimation, playing Russian Roulette with his life.

"Incredible" was Dyer's word for what Jerry had been able to accomplish under dialysis and after transplant: full teaching load, travel, and performing. Dyer had seen other patients who'd done amazing things but not patients with Jerry's combined medical problems. How could he warn Jerry without ruining his outlook? Dyer decided that he could only give his best advice and let Jerry take it from there.

He advised Jerry and Dottie that Jerry was overdoing, that he had a new kidney, but an old problem. He still had diabetes, which restricts blood flow to the capillaries and causes blindness, kidney failure, high blood pressure, stroke and heart attack. The transplant corrected one of the effects of diabetes, but it couldn't correct diabetes.

Dr. Filo also advised caution: "Watch Jerry's blood pressure; we don't want him to have a stroke."

A March 1985 concert in El Cajon, California, proved the truth in both doctors' words.

It had been a long trip and a restless night in strange surroundings. Jerry was not feeling very peppy when he stood to play in the El Cajon Wesleyan Church on Sunday morning. He'd hardly begun to play "The Carnival of Venice" when Dottie knew something was wrong. He was playing like a beginning fifth-grader, with squawky sounds, slurred transitions and non-existent tonguing.

Fear knotted Dottie's stomach. A stroke, that's what it must be. The doctors had warned of the possibility of strokes and heart attacks. Dottie's gaze went to Jeff and Marcy, who were seated to her left on the platform. Marcy's face was stricken, Jeff's eyes were dark with worry. Mom, do something! their eyes said.

Dottie, close to Jerry, touched his arm and said softly, "Jerry, you have to sit down now." She pulled on his sleeve. "Jerry?"

But Jerry, slumped, looking like an actor in a silent movie, was moving his fingers on the valves, but there was no sound coming out of the horn – a trumpet of clay.

There was silence, too, in the sanctuary. The congregation was giving all their energy in sympathy for the struggling performer before them.

Jeff, at the back of the band with his drums, hissed

at Marcy. "Get Dad!"

Marcy could not move.

Then Jeff directed his words to Dottie. "Make him stop, make him sit down." He did not want those strangers staring at his dad.

"I can't," Dottie whispered back.

Finally, at the end of the number, Jeff worked his way around chairs and instruments and taking his dad's arm, helped lower him to a chair.

"No, I can do it," said Jerry. "I can go on."

Marcy, who could see the left side of Jerry's face, the drooping eye and cheek, could stand no more. She bent over the horn on her lap and wept.

Jeff and Dottie convinced Jerry to remain seated. Then Dottie, the announcer for the concert, stood, and with a levity she didn't feel, said, "You know these transplants, they kick up sometimes." She proceeded to offer Jerry's testimony, giving him a few minutes to rest.

After the concert, the extent of the stroke damage was clear to all but Jerry. His whole left side showed evidence of the stroke: drooping face, limp arm and dragging foot.

"You've had a stroke, Jerry," said Dottie.

"No, I'm fine," answered Jerry.

"Shouldn't we go to the hospital, Mom?"

"No, I'm fine," Jerry repeated. "I'll be better if I eat. All I need is a little sugar."

The difficulty with which Jerry ate further belied the damage of the stroke and increased the concern of his family. They called Dr. Filo in Indiana.

"Yes, he's probably had a stroke," said the doctor, "but if he's still on his feet and going, there's no need to go to the hospital. There probably wouldn't be any sign of it anyway. Let him rest and take it easy, and I'll see him when you get back."

"There, see!" said Jerry when he'd heard what the doctor had said. "He said 'probably'. I'll be all right, it's just the long trip and no sleep last night. I'll just rest this afternoon."

Jerry's family was frightened. They'd seen his reaction to blindness, kidney failure and transplant, but they'd never seen the denial he was exhibiting with the stroke. Though he couldn't see the stroke's effect on his face, surely he could feel that liquid did not stay in his mouth, that his left arm was immobile and his left foot was dragging. Maybe the stroke had damaged his thinking process.

Jerry *was* having trouble thinking clearly. He was so tired, so "out of it" that he wasn't aware that he was dragging a foot or slurring his words. When he reached his host's home, Dottie took him immediately to his room where Jerry sat on the bed, rolled his feet from the floor and stretched out on the bed. He was so tired and weak, numb even. But, he decided, it was just jet lag, the lack of sleep the night before. He would be fine after a nap.

The nap didn't make a startling difference. He moved in a mental vagueness that accepted only fatigue and the knowledge that he *had* to be fine because there were still 16 days of tour left.

When he warmed up on his horn that evening, he found that he'd lost feeling in his mouth, which prevented him from using his embouchure properly.

But it was three days later before Jerry would admit that he'd had a stroke. At a band prayer session before the evening performance, his worried family and students included him in their supplications.

"Please, Lord, help Jerry. Guide his understanding and heal him."

Then, slowly, haltingly, with a slight lisp to the words, Jerry's voice fell on the quiet room. "I guess I did lose the left side of my embouchure . . ."

The embouchure was to remain "lost" for months into the future, recaptured only after paralyzing fear and intense practice.

Chapter 10

The Lord Can Give You Peace

Friday March 7, 1986. 5:00 a.m.

Dottie sat up, shut off the alarm and shook Jerry.

"Time to get up, Honey. It's clinic day!"

In the kitchen, she put the teakettle on the stove, grabbed a cup and tea bag from the cupboard and took a peek at the frosty backyard. Just a few icy spots where rain had settled. Jerry and Stan Storey, president of Dimensions in Brass, should have no trouble getting to Indianapolis.

She reviewed the schedule for the day. She would be teaching, of course, and Jerry would have one of his "hurry up and wait" days. He would leave home by 6:15, arrive at the I.U. Med Center in Indianapolis between 7:30 and 7:45, have his blood drawn and then wait until 1:30 or 2:00 to get the results of the tests. A routine Friday.

But clinic days could never be taken for granted. Twice before, in November of 1983 and November of 1984, Jerry had gone to clinic feeling good, with no thought of trouble, and had been admitted to the hospital because his creatinine level was too high.

They could never tell what forces were at work in the "subterranean" chambers of Jerry's body. Diabetes was like a quiet mole going about his work and then surfacing at some unexpected spot. Except that when he surfaced, he suddenly grew to a towering monster, his eyeless orifices gleaming with fire and his clawed feet striking at them, tearing at their comfortable routines and destroying their peace.

Diabetes, unlike the mole that cleared tunnels, laid masses of material in the hair-like capillaries of the body, barring the flow of blood. The eyes and kidneys, which contained the greatest numbers of these minute tunnels, were affected first. But one by one, the limbs, brain and heart sustained damage.

The other forces at work in Jerry's body were the white corpuscles. The national guard of the body, they rushed reserves wherever there was need and carried on an unceasing campaign to drive out alien cells and organs. In other words, Jerry's kidney!

But why borrow trouble? Dottie thought. Things were going well. Jerry was gradually regaining his playing skills after the damage of the stroke; Dottie, a proud '84 *magna cum laude* graduate of Marion College, was teaching first grade at Francis Slocum School in Marion, and the clinic visits had been reduced to one every eight weeks. A comfortable schedule – life was good.

Dottie took a sip of her tea. In fact, things had been going so well that she seldom went with Jerry to clinic anymore. Stan was taking Jerry to Indianapolis today, *if* she got busy and got his breakfast. She hurried from the kitchen.

"Jerry, will you be ready to eat in about 15 minutes?"

By 8:30, Jerry had had blood drawn, exchanged salutations and news with the staff on duty, and settled into the small waiting room in the I.U. Med Center's fourth-floor renal transplant area.

The morning went quickly. Jerry and Stan visited with the patients as they came and went, sharing experiences and comparing "numbers." Potassium, calcium and phosphorus, hematocrit, BUN and creatinine were the blood components measured on clinic days. But it was the BUN and creatinine that patients watched with a wary eye. If the BUN, the level of protein wastes in the blood, was over 100, uremic symptoms could set in. If the creatinine, the level of wastes in the blood, was ten, it was cause for alarm.

The numbers had sent Jerry to the hospital two times before. While he was in the hospital, it was the numbers that ruled his life and the lives of other patients as they lay on their beds, submitting to IVs of drugs that made them weak, irritable and dopey.

Patients lived for the daily posting of numbers on the charts outside their doors. When someone walked by, silence reigned. Was that someone bringing the numbers? Were the numbers going down? Would they be able to go home soon?

When interns finally entered results on the charts, patients and their families waited until the pad-pad of footsteps had faded away and then went to see whether the ATG and Medrol were quieting the body's battle with the kidney. When the numbers were good, patients rejoiced with one another; when they were bad, they grieved together.

But it had been a year and a half since there had been any problem. Jerry, who always tried to think positively, turned his thoughts to something that happened a few weeks before, on their last trip to Indianapolis. It hadn't been a trip to the hospital, but rather a Dimensions in Brass performance at the Principals' Convention at the Adams Mark Hotel. Their increasingly unreliable bus had produced so much smoke that it had set off the smoke alarm in the hotel parking garage. Jerry smiled to himself. Then, after the Dimensions had played for the convention, Governor Orr had risen to speak and, seeing Jerry's "playpen," had asked if he could stand in Jerry's "litter box." Dimensions in Brass performances provided plenty of memories for Jerry to smile about.

At 1:30, after eating lunch and stocking up on medications, Jerry returned to Renal Transplant and picked up his chart. Stan read the numbers aloud and Jerry's heart hit bottom. Oh no! He was in trouble. The chemistries were a mess. What could have caused such a drastic change?

He'd been taking Minoxidil and had been retaining fluid because of it. Was the Minoxidil causing other problems? Or was the kidney failure the cause of the fluid retention? When Jerry talked to the doctor, he wasn't surprised to hear that he was to be admitted to the hospital.

By the next day, Jerry's condition had worsened. His creatinine level went up; his creatinine clearance, which indicates kidney function, dropped alarmingly to 11, one point above the number at which the kidney is usually removed! Jerry's routine check-up, his comfortable schedule had been violently interrupted again. The miraculous, life-sustaining antibodies, the national guard of his body, were causing the death of an organ he needed to have to survive.

As the days passed, the loss of the kidney became more and more imminent. Doctors were scrambling, plumbing their knowledge, for a way to avoid removing the kidney. There was a chance, they decided, that, since Jerry's blood pressure was so high, his renal artery was blocked. It might help to do surgery and free the artery. But first they would have to do an arteriogram.

Jerry rebelled. "I don't want to do that!" he said.

Jerry had been cut and jabbed for three and a half years. He'd joked through a shunt and fistula; he'd kept a stiff upper lip with surgery and the innumerable blood tests, but another arteriogram was insupportable.

"I don't want to do this," he said.

There was silence in the room. The doctors exchanged glances. Jerry was usually cooperative, cheerful.

"The surgery?" asked Dr. Filo.

"The arteriogram," said Jerry. "Isn't there something else we can do?"

"Well, we really should get a picture of the situation before we decide to do surgery . . . with an arteriogram we just thread a catheter in through your groin and . . ."

Jerry knew what they did. He'd had it done after the transplant. The surgeon had inserted and inserted and inserted the large needle, Jerry's pain and tension growing with each attempt. Afterward, the opening had not healed and he'd bled for 12 hours. Like that opening in the groin had been, the memory was a raw wound, a returning nightmare that he didn't want repeated. And besides, something told him that the problem was not in the renal artery.

"I don't want to do this," Jerry said again. "Isn't there something else we can do? They messed it up the last time."

Dr. Filo spoke carefully. "I don't see any way around this, Jerry. We have to look at all the alternatives before we consider removing the kidney."

Jerry's fear and dread built, prompting him to vocalize his feelings to the surgeon in charge of the arteriogram.

"I'm really upset about this. They messed it up the

last time . . ." and he recounted his previous experience.

"Well, there's no excuse for that," said the doctor. "The veins of a diabetic are hard to find, but I assure you that what happened before won't happen this time."

Jerry was relieved to find that it didn't happen again. The procedure was quick and relatively painless, but when Filo and Leapman visited with Jerry later, there was good news and bad news.

"The good news, Jerry, is that the artery isn't blocked. The bad news is that it looks like we're going to have to take out the kidney."

A sinking inside, that was the feeling. Like his heart and stomach had fallen out of place. Take out the kidney . . . more surgery, weeks of recuperation and then back on dialysis. Months and years on dialysis.

But what else could he do? It was start again or die. After the doctors left, Jerry reached for the phone and dialed his office at Marion College. He told Marcy the problem and asked her to call her mother and then spoke to one of the members of the Dimensions in Brass.

"Hey look, will you guys pray for me? I don't want to lose this kidney."

The staff at Francis Slocum School were concerned about Dottie. Another crisis. How could she stand up under all the pressure? Dottie answered, "I can handle it," arranged for a substitute, picked up clothes and Marcy and headed to Indianapolis.

When Jerry had called two days before to say that Filo had admitted him to the hospital, it had been "business as usual" for Dottie. Transplant patients were admitted to the hospital all the time, given ATG and Medrol to stabilize the kidney and then released. Jerry himself had had three rejections. Why be surprised when a condition produced expected emergencies?

But the news that there was no artery blockage was a blow to Dottie. She'd been so sure, so positive everything would be OK, that Jerry would receive Solu-Medrol to quiet the antibodies working on the kidney and be out of the hospital within a week.

A week! Now he'd be in the hospital at least a month and when he came out he would be weakened from surgery before he even went on the dialysis that made him feel so bad.

A great darkness settled over Dottie's spirit. It was

as if she were in a deep hole and the earth had fallen in on top of her. I can't! she thought. I can't go through it again. It's too much!

At Francis Slocum School, Dottie received a page in her room.

"Phone call, Dottie. It's Marcy."

"OK, thank you." Dottie called back.

Dottie went to the office and picked up the phone. "Hello?" she said.

"Mom-m!" Marcy's choked voice began. And then she wept, out of control.

"OK, Honey, OK. It's going to be all right. Take a deep breath and tell me what's happened."

Amid the sounds of sniffles and tortured breaths, there came, "It's Dad . . . he says . . . they're going to have to take out . . . The Kidney!" and she wept again.

Dottie felt as if she'd been hit in the stomach. Take out the kidney!

"Mom?"

"Yes, Honey?"

"Mom, what will we do?"

Dottie, who always tried to act the way she wanted to feel, answered, "We'll pray about it. I'll see you after school, Honey, and we'll go down to Indianapolis."

It had been too much before! Six years of summoning up all the strength and hope she had so that she could encourage Jerry. She could see those days, hear the buzzers, smell the Clorox and cleaning solutions, and feel the emotions and fatigue. The knowledge was like all of those days had been condensed and placed on her shoulders at once.

Before, the crises had come one at a time. Now there was no ignorance, no numbness. She knew the route, could see the terrible terrain of dialysis. She'd be chained, just like Jerry, jerked and dragged by that machine and its pulsing tubes and rasping buzzers, when she was already committed to a busy schedule of teaching. When they'd done dialysis before, she'd been taking classes, arranged around the dialysis. But now she was teaching – and she needed to teach! – how could she work all day and do dialysis too? *When* would they do dialysis?

She would be tired, Jerry would be tired, maybe too tired this time, maybe . . . No! No! Why is he doing this to me? I can't go through this again!

Jerry was struggling too. Dialysis was like slogging through mile after mile of heavy sand, dragging step after step to the top of a rise, only to find that the sand hills stretched clear to the farthest horizon.

And what about Dottie? She was in it with him. Pulling and encouraging, running the machine. Working on a degree and then teaching so she could help financially. She hadn't done anything to deserve this.

Jerry slipped deeper and deeper into thought. The questions were a broken record in his brain, repeating in mid-sentence when he awoke briefly at night. How could they manage financially? He wouldn't be able to teach and travel as much. How could he do it *physically?* Before, he'd just wanted to stay in bed, but he'd dragged himself out and kept going. Would he be able to go at all this time, what with going on dialysis right after surgery? He hated it – the emotion knotted him inside – hated it for Dottie, and for himself. How could they do it all over again?

Jerry and Dottie, in spite of their natural resilience and positive outlooks, had finally sustained a blow that sent them reeling. They withdrew into thought. There was perfunctory talk about IVs or get-well greetings, but most of the time Jerry listened to the TV and Dottie walked the hall or, with a book open before her, retreated into thought again.

Strong emotions collided in Dottie: anger, love, sympathy, guilt. She knew Jerry was feeling guilty, so she felt doubly guilty because he was feeling bad and she couldn't reassure him. As a result of these thoughts and feelings, there came the need to work off her tension, so she walked again.

Meanwhile, at Marion College, the Dimensions in Brass students had organized a prayer marathon. Between classes, before lunch, at 2:00 a.m., at 4:35 a.m., all around the clock, students prayed for Jerry and his kidney, lifting up in intercessory prayer the struggling body and emotions of Jerry Franks and his family.

Dottie, on the other hand, was having trouble praying. She knew she should, but she couldn't form words, couldn't reach through the barrier of hopelessness and self-pity to draw strength from the Lord.

Dottie recognized it as self-pity, the emotion that the books had called the primary cause of depression. Was that why she couldn't call out to the Lord? Was she too ashamed? Would He condemn her for not being able to pray?

No. Dottie was quieted, at peace, as understanding came to her. The Lord had created her and all her feelings. He knew that she would feel this way, so He'd even provided for the times when she couldn't pray: intercessory prayer.

She'd been unable to pray once before in Jerry's illness. It had been that black night five years ago when Jerry's kidneys had first failed. Lying on her black couch with her black thoughts, she'd been too numb and weak. Then there had come an awareness, an understanding. It was all right if she couldn't pray, because others were praying for her and their prayers were enough.

Bursting with love and gratitude, Dottie had wept. What a wonder, what a knowledge. God loved her so much that He'd even provided for the times when grief and discouragement rendered her incapable of praying.

Tears washed over Dottie's cheeks as she remembered. People were praying for her now too: their families, their church, Jerry's students, her friends at Francis Slocum. Like a storm blown away by a gentle, fresh wind, Dottie's despair drifted away. The Lord loved her, He would help her. All she needed was a willingness to go through dialysis again and God would help her handle it.

Poor Jerry, Dottie thought suddenly. How he must feel! She had not shouted recriminations at him, but she'd been so quiet, so wrapped up in herself that he surely knew what she was thinking. She needed to tell him how she felt now.

Dottie left off pacing the hospital halls and made her way to Jerry's room where she was suddenly shy, conscience-stricken over her behavior and thoughts. Jerry was the one who'd been cut and poked, exhausted by dialysis; but he had struggled to keep going, to meet his obligations to his family. How could she forget that? How could she get so tied up in herself that she forgot that?

She took a tentative step into the room. "Jerry? . . ."

"Dottie? Hi!" said Jerry.

She walked to the side of the bed that was free of tubes.

"Jerry, I have to tell you something." She put her

hand over his.

"OK."

"Jerry, it's all right, we'll get through it." She spoke quickly. "I've decided that we'll dialyze in the evening. It might mean that we'll get to bed late, but we can do it."

Jerry squeezed her hand. His voice tight with emotion, he said, "I'm sorry, Dottie. I hate it . . ." He drew a tortured breath and began to cry.

Dottie, unable to speak, bent over Jerry, wrapping her arms under him and laying her tear-damp cheek on his shoulder. Once again she was in tune with her husband, hurting when he hurt, weeping at his weeping.

"It's all right, Honey. It will be all right."

Jerry wiped at his cheek with the IV-encumbered hand. "I've been lying here thinking, wondering how we could do it again . . . how I could put you through that again . . ." Emotion choked off the words.

"We'll be all right, Honey." She hugged him tight. With his free hand, Jerry held her close. "The Lord will help us. It'll be all right."

One year later, March 18, 1987, Jerry sat on the platform in the Great Hall of the Hubert Humphrey Building in Washington, D.C. To his right was Vice President Bush and Rose Bowen. To his left sat Dottie, and beyond her, the black-uniformed Dimensions in Brass, their golden instruments resting in their laps. At the podium Dr. Otis Bowen was making some opening remarks.

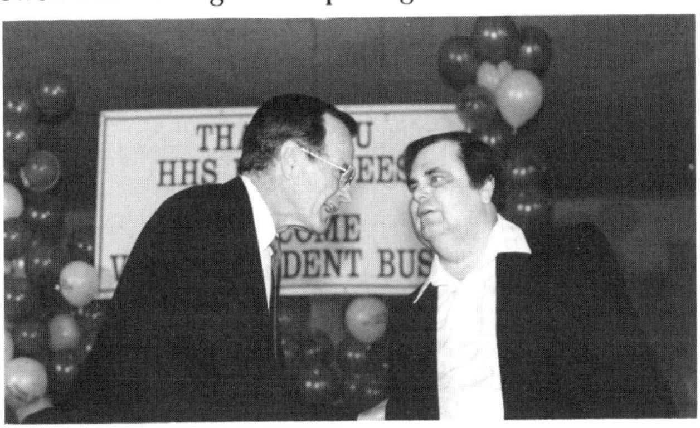

Vice President, George Bush greeting Jerry at the Health and Human Services luncheon in Washington, D.C. (1987)

Bowen, the Secretary of Health and Human Services, having heard that Jerry would be in the Washington area, had requested that the Dimensions in Brass perform for a luncheon in honor of his staff, whom Bowen esteems highly for their compassionate work with the people they serve. The luncheon had a picnic theme, complete with decorations, Indiana tulips, and banners welcoming Bush.

"And," continued Bowen, "I wanted to express our thanks to all of you for your help over the last 18 months . . . and to introduce some of our guests this afternoon: Sam Pierce, the Secretary of Housing and Urban Development, Jerry Franks, and the Dimensions in Brass . . . he and his fine group will be playing for us later on . . ."

Jerry gave Dottie's hand a squeeze and thought back to the beginning of the Dimensions in Brass. Eleven kids, practicing wherever they could in Byer Hall. Eleven kids, an organization he'd dedicated to the Lord. He'd prayed that it might be unique in Christian music. His prayers had been answered.

He'd promised the Lord that if he could get professional training and experience he would teach Christian young people. He'd kept his promise. But not by himself.

In everything, at every turn, God had done what no one else could do, showing His power in ways that there could be no doubt who had accomplished the feat.

Back in 1966, when Jerry had decided to go to Grace, he'd been approached by an agent. "Hey, Man!" he'd said, "you shouldn't go to that hick town. Let me handle your career and I'll have you on the stage of the Midwest National Band Clinic before you're 30!" Jerry hadn't signed with the agent, but he had appeared at the Midwest National Band Clinic. God had beat the agent's timetable and had helped him, Jerry Franks, a teacher-band director from a small Christian college, to appear at Dodger Stadium and in Washington, D.C.

God had reversed the natural effects of blindness, allowing him to play and direct when doctors said he shouldn't be able to. Who but God could give him the spirit and strength to keep going under dialysis? Who but God, one year earlier, March of 1986, could have helped his body make peace with his donated kidney, when doctors were ready to remove the organ?

No one but God! God was the creator of his talent and his ability to devise and invent. And God was the creator of his good wife Dottie. The lump returned to Jerry's throat as he thought of Dottie.

When he'd had kidney failure, Dottie had learned to drive a car though she hated everything mechanical. Jerry suppressed a smile at the memory of a question she'd once asked. After 39 years of riding in a car, she'd asked what the two pedals on the floor were for. Rob had always said that Dottie could never be accused of "joy riding" because she hated to drive.

Only God could have given him such a wife, who didn't fail him when the going was not just rough, but virtually impossible. At every juncture, Dottie had come through. She'd pinpointed the reason for his depression the summer before his transplant and had studied books and asked questions until she'd ascertained that Seconal was the cause, and she had seen to it that he was taken off harmful medications.

She'd performed the tedious, stressful duties of dialysis over 300 times in two years and she hadn't yelled at him about what his illness had done to her. She hadn't failed him when she was at her lowest point the year before. She'd said, "It's all right, we'll get through it."

And now here he was. On tour again. God surely did work things out in a magnificent way (Jerry thought of the day before), even when you were reluctant and grumbling.

In Washington the day before, he, his family and the Dimensions had had to cut short their sightseeing to fulfill an engagement in the Baltimore Wesleyan Church. Jerry had not received confirmation of the appearance, so in addition to their reluctance to leave off sightseeing and their concern about getting a good night's rest, the students had been upset about a "wild goose chase with no audience at the other end." The complaining was epidemic. Even the most positive joined in.

"Well, I think we should go back to Washington!"

"Yeah. You couldn't even reach the pastor when you called. There's probably no one there."

"Oh, for Pete's sake! What are we doing now? Asking another bus driver for directions?"

"The church must be in Outer Mongolia."

"Not Mongolia. Have you looked out the window? Looks more like a red light district to me."

"Look. Winos! Are you sure we're going in the right direction?"

A second stop to call the pastor had produced no results, but the bus, rumbling and coughing and adding to the students' feelings of uneasiness, had moved slowly onward, finally coming to a stop before a small church in a very bad area of the town.

"I'll bet we get mugged!"

"Doesn't look inhabited to me. Let's go back."

But the pastor had been there, *and* his aging parishioners, *and* all the resplendent preparations imaginable: beautifully decorated hall, tables and cakes. Banners proclaimed: "Welcome Dimensions in Brass."

It had been like walking from Kansas to Oz, from darkness to light, to enter that church. The attitudes of the young musicians had been transformed too. After getting acquainted with the people and circumstances of the small church, they had been guilt-stricken.

Here was a congregation of 25 people who couldn't afford both food and an offering for the Dimensions in Brass, so they'd obtained donations from businessmen. They didn't have many members, so they'd gone door-to-door, distributing leaflets and inviting people to attend the concert. They'd raised a $250.00 offering for the band. "They've never done anything this big before," the happy pastor reported.

"Big" described the blessing of the service. Band members had entered with a grumbling spirit and received the special blessings of giving spirits – the Holy Spirit living in the good people of that church.

"They can't afford to give us that $250.00," said one student. "Can't we give it back?"

"No," said another, "that would be like a slap in the face to them."

Stan Storey commented, "You know, we thought we needed a good night's rest, but the Lord knew we needed the Baltimore church."

Jerry's thoughts returned to the present as Dr. Bowen's voice rose. "Ladies and gentlemen, Jerry Franks!"

Jerry stood and, with his left hand on Dottie's shoulder, shuffled to the box in front of the band. After a series of numbers, he turned to the audience and told his story.

"Easter Morning of 1978 I awoke blind. But I've been a Christian ever since I was a little boy, so I prayed that day, 'Lord, Help!' And a peace came over my soul. One hour after I went blind, I did my first concert and then went on to Iowa and did 25 more.

"The doctor told me all the things I couldn't do: I couldn't play, go on stage or conduct. After he got done, I said, 'I wish you'd told me that two weeks ago; I've already done 25 concerts.'

"The doctor didn't know what to say. Fact is, he had even suggested that I come to Washington, D.C. He said in Washington, D.C., they've got a program for blind people where you can set up a hamburger stand and sell hamburgers on the Capitol lawn. I said, 'You've got to be kidding! I'd eat up all the profits!'

"So I decided to go on, but the diabetes wasn't finished with me yet. About six years ago I was rushed to the hospital with kidney failure, but with the help of some good doctors, I pulled out. For the next two years I was on kidney dialysis. Then about four years ago I got a transplant and it was successful. Boy, it was great to just be blind again!

"But that hasn't been easy either, 'cause I've had three major rejections, and with the last one, a year ago, they said the kidney would have to come out. But the Lord was with me; the kidney miraculously turned around and here I stand today."

Jerry paused, then quietly went on, "I don't know what problems you might have today. We've all got them, but I'm just here to tell you that we've got a great God that can take care of any problem you might have, and all you have to do is tell Him."

God can use even a trumpet of clay to play for His glory.

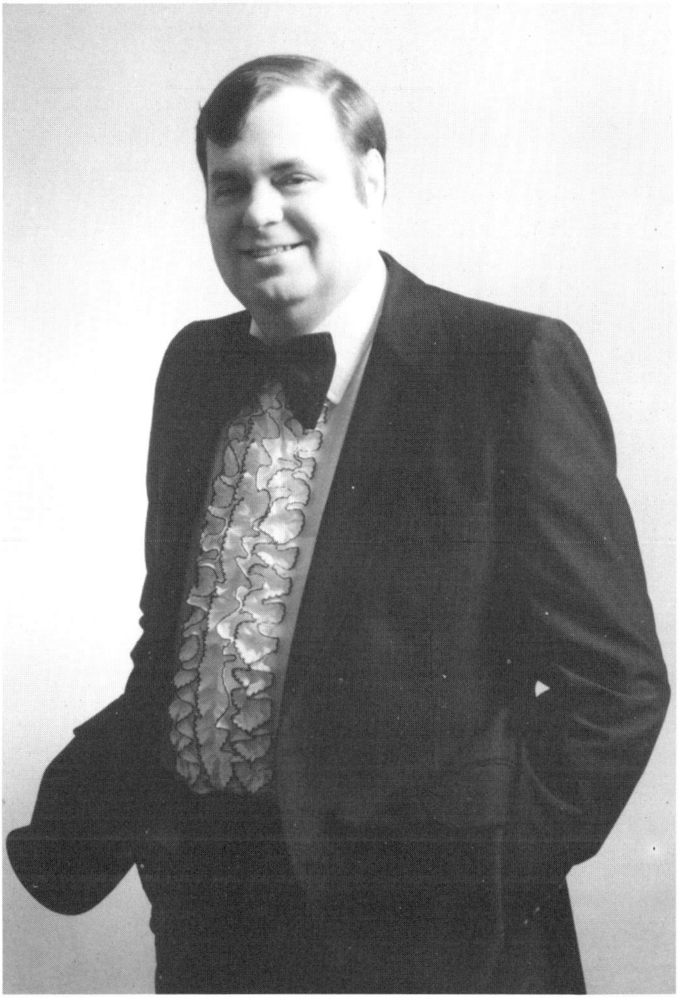

Jerry Franks

And whatever ye shall ask in my name, that will I do, that the Father may be glorified in the Son (John 14:13).